Your
Pregnancy

YOUR

Pregnancy

Reassuring Answers to the Questions of Mothers-to-Be

• • •

RONALD M. CAPLAN, M.D.,
WITH BETTY ROTHBART

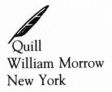

Quill
William Morrow
New York

It is the policy of William Morrow and Company, Inc., and its imprints and affiliates, recognizing the importance of preserving what has been written, to print the books we publish on acid-free paper, and we exert our best efforts to that end.

Library of Congress Cataloging-in-Publication Data

Caplan, Ronald M.
    Your pregnancy : reassuring answers to the questions of mothers-
to-be / Ronald M. Caplan with Betty Rothbart.
        p.   cm.
    Includes index.
    ISBN 0-688-10826-1
    1. Pregnancy—Miscellanea.   I. Rothbart, Betty.   II. Title.
RG525.C342   1992
618.2'4—dc20   92-14145
                                                               CIP

Printed in the United States of America

First Quill Edition

1 2 3 4 5 6 7 8 9 10

BOOK DESIGN BY PATRICE FODERO

ILLUSTRATIONS © 1992 BY DOLORES R. SANTOLIQUIDO

Acknowledgments

Many thanks to Debra Grant, R.N., Fellow of the American College of Childbirth Educators; our editor, Andy Dutter; and our agent, Wendy Lipkind, for their insights and encouragement.

Contents

Introduction

At last, after Gloria had labored for hours, with her husband John by her side, childbirth began. First, slowly, out pushed the baby's head, his eyes squeezed tightly shut. One shoulder nudged forward, then the other, and finally, in one determined wriggle, all the rest of him followed.

John exclaimed, "He's so big!"

Gloria, amazed, said, "It's a baby!"

As soon as she spoke, she realized the absurdity of her words. Of course it was a baby! What else would it be? But in fact, this was the first moment in nine months that she truly connected her pregnancy to the birth of an actual person—her son, Michael.

Such is the intensity of the pregnancy experience. Your silhouette changes, and you feel amazing sensations; perhaps, like many women, you "speak" to the fetus, caress your growing abdomen, choose a boy's name and a girl's—yet somehow you are still dubious that the roundness of your belly will translate into a ten-fingers, ten-toes baby at the end of nine months. But it will; within you a life is budding, and you are its world.

Pregnancy is like switching from a regular bicycle to a tandem bike: For the first time, you have a rider who depends on you to map out a route, steer carefully, and arrive unharmed. When you first embark on the pregnancy journey, the nine months stretch before you like terrain that is well traveled—but not yet by you. So it may seem tantalizing, but perhaps a bit scary, too.

Other women's tales probably affect your outlook. What have you heard? Some women relate pregnancy war stories: "I was sick all the time, my feet swelled, I gained too much weight, I didn't feel like making love, I was depressed, I was worried, and the labor-room nurse scolded me." Just what you need to hear!

Or maybe you've heard a somewhat sunnier perspective: "Sure, I had morning sickness in the first trimester, but knowing I was pregnant made it tolerable. By the second trimester, I was more energetic than ever. I loved getting big and feeling the baby move inside me. My husband was so tender. Labor was intense, but watching the baby come out was the highlight of my life."

Every woman has her own story; now you will have yours. Though pregnancy has its share of discomforts and concerns, the aim of this book is to provide you with not only a detailed map for your journey, but also the reassurances that can help make your experience a positive one.

Want to hear the most hilarious medical phrase? It's when a practitioner solemnly describes a healthy pregnancy as "uneventful." *Every* pregnancy is eventful. New developments occur continuously. And they culminate in what is unquestionably the most thrilling event in the world, the emergence of a new life.

Some pregnancy events, however, can be intensely unnerving. Not only are your hormones playing new tunes inside you; all of a sudden you hear one of the world's most cacophonous choruses: the famed "Advice on How to Have a Baby." If you've been pregnant longer than two minutes, you have probably already heard enough warnings and "shoulds" to fill a Pentagon manual. A pregnant woman is a magnet for advice, much of it conflicting and unasked-for. Everyone has an opinion—your neighbor, your boss, your friends, your mother, and your mother-in-law. Even perfect strangers get into the act, like the lady in the supermarket who advises you to put back the cucumbers and subsist solely on yams.

The advice can be terribly confusing, and it can make pregnancy more stressful than it needs to be. For some reason, advice-givers seem to have a personal investment in winning you over to their point of view. Almost as if they got a commission with each new convert.

Consider, for example, the low-tech camp and the high-tech camp. Each will battle to win you over to its "politically correct" side. *Always* use a midwife/*never* use one. *Always* breast-feed/*always* bottle-feed. *Always* avoid painkillers during labor/*never* go without them. The advice chorus croons on and on. In this song, you always hear the long version.

It is important to know both low-tech and high-tech alternatives, but finally you must make decisions based on your own values, preferences, and instincts. Let the following statement guide you: *Pregnancy's one and only goal is to give mother and baby the greatest chance of being and staying healthy from conception through birth.* Keeping that in mind can help you complete your pregnancy with health, sanity, and sense of humor intact.

And then you will be ready for an even *more* adventurous journey: motherhood. The beauty of pregnancy is that you get nine months to adjust to literally sharing your innermost self with another human being, a relationship that is like no other. Your relationship with your child will last a lifetime. Give it the best start you can, and enjoy the miracle of creating new life.

Your
Pregnancy

CHAPTER 1

In the Beginning

Q: What are the signs of pregnancy?

The signs may be as subtle as your breasts feeling slightly heavier, or as obtrusive as morning sickness or frequent urination. For most women, a missed menstrual period is the first clue.

The tricky thing is, each of these signs might not really indicate pregnancy. Heavy breasts may mean menstruation is imminent or be associated with premenstrual syndrome. Vomiting and nausea may signal stress, food poisoning, or other diseases. Frequent urination is also a sign of urinary-tract infection or anxiety. And a missed period may result from recent weight loss, illness, stress, or exhaustion. Even travel can be the culprit, since the body sometimes takes weeks to adjust to time and schedule changes.

Q: When and how can I find out for sure that I am pregnant?

It depends on how soon you want to know. If you can't get to a doctor's office, go to the drugstore and buy a home pregnancy test. Like urine tests done in a laboratory, home pregnancy tests discover whether your urine contains hCG (human chorionic gonadotropin), a pregnancy hormone.

You may enjoy learning the news in the privacy of your own home. But home pregnancy tests (and lab urine tests) can yield false positive or false negative results if urine is tested too soon after conception, if the test is done incorrectly, if the urine sample is accidentally contaminated, or if the test is defective.

Therefore it is a good idea to confirm pregnancy through a blood test, also called a *serum pregnancy test*. Blood tests offer greater accuracy than urine tests. And they not only detect hCG; they measure it. Too much or too little hCG can alert your doctor to potential problems such as miscarriage or ectopic pregnancy, a dangerous condition in which the pregnancy occurs in a Fallopian tube instead of the uterus.

A pelvic exam conducted by a doctor is reliable confirmation of pregnancy—and a first step in prenatal care.

Q: How do I choose a doctor—or should I choose a nurse-midwife?

For normal pregnancies where everything goes smoothly, either a doctor or a certified nurse-midwife can give you the care you need. Some women believe that a midwife will avoid unnecessary medical interventions and invite a closer rapport. Yet that viewpoint does not acknowledge that physicians and midwives are individuals. Some are warmer and more patient than others, some are quicker to intervene medically than others.

Of course, it is important to feel comfortable with your practitioner. But nine months of rapport add up to nothing compared with one crucial minute during childbirth when you might hemorrhage and only a physician can help you. However capable and supportive a midwife may be, she simply cannot handle every complication that may arise. And complications do happen, often unexpectedly, even to healthy and normal women and babies. It makes sense to select an experienced physician who can give you and your baby the advantage of medical technology if you need it.

Some physicians have certified nurse-midwives on their staff who conduct routine examinations, answer questions, teach childbirth classes, and assist with childbirth.

Q: Should I plan to give birth at a hospital, at home, or at a birthing center?

You are right to consider this question early in your pregnancy, because you want to select a practitioner who will honor your choice. It became fashionable for a time to consider giving birth at home or at a birthing center not connected to a hospital. Both options may offer a warmer ambience than a hospital, and a perfectly normal birth in either setting can be a lovely experience.

Yet choosing to give birth at home or at a freestanding birthing center a distance from a hospital could prove to be a tragic decision. The most ordinary pregnancy can have the most dramatic outcome. No one can ever know in advance which mother may hemorrhage, or need an emergency cesarean section, or oxygen, or other aid. Nor can anyone predict which baby may need immediate intensive perinatal care. If an emergency occurs in a hospital, medical specialists, equipment, an intensive-care ward, and a neonatal intensive-care unit (available in a Level III hospital) are right there. But if you are at home or in a freestanding birthing center, just consider the harrowing logistics. The emergency call to 911. Waiting for the ambulance to come. The drive to the hospital, perhaps through heavy traffic, during which bleeding may continue unchecked. The arrival at the hospital and further delay until the right medical personnel can be located, scrubbed, and ready to help you. Precious seconds and minutes elapse, time that may be critical for the health and survival of yourself and your child.

It is not worth the risk. Pregnancy and labor are dynamic, continuously evolving processes, with physiologic changes to both mother and child. Boost the odds for enabling you and your baby to be healthy and together for a lifetime by giving birth in a hospital, a setting that is equipped to handle any last-minute, health-or life-threatening changes.

Women originally gave birth at home because they had no

other options, or because in bygone days hospitals were hotbeds of infection, and home birth was safer. Neither of those conditions still holds. Women who lost babies in home births because they could not get to the hospital in time would never counsel anyone else to choose home birth over hospital birth. Take advantage of the fact that you are living in a country and time when medical technology works miracles with fragile newborns and their mothers.

Some women want to give birth at home because of concern about insensitive or outdated hospital policies, such as those that forbid the baby's father to be present at delivery or that require women to lie flat on their backs during labor instead of being able to move around freely. Today, however, many if not all hospitals encourage the father to participate in labor and childbirth and have more enlightened policies about such concerns as labor, prepping, and infant rooming-in. Many hospitals offer homelike birthing rooms that feature soft music, rocking chairs, birthing beds, appealing posters, and other amenities. There, you and your partner can be together throughout labor and childbirth, and cuddle your newborn infant.

When choosing a practitioner, always consider the hospital with which he or she is affiliated. Find out the hospital's policies and ask whether you can request waivers from any policies with which you disagree. Write to hospitals you reject and tell them why. That is one reason policies change: when they result in the loss of customers.

Q: *When is my due date?*
If you know when you conceived, just add 267 days to that date. But most women do not know the date of conception. Therefore, calculate the *probable* date of ovulation and conception by adding 280 days (40 weeks) to the day your last menstrual period began. So if your last period was on January 1, the theoretical pregnancy starting date was January 15; 280 days from January 1 gives you an October 8 due date.

Or use "Nägele's rule." From the first day of your last period, subtract three months, then add seven days. To continue with the above example, three months earlier than January 1 is October 1. Plus seven days produces the October 8 due date.

Most practitioners have a pregnancy wheel, a nifty gadget that tells you your due date instantly.

These methods of estimating the due date are most reliable for women who have regular twenty-eight-day menstrual cycles. Other clues to how long you have been pregnant are the size of your uterus, how soon the fetal heartbeat is heard, and when you first feel the baby move. In many cases, an early sonogram may be necessary to ascertain the fetus's gestational age.

Remember that a due date is only approximate. Babies have a way of lingering longer in that nice warm amniotic fluid, or of getting bored with all that tranquillity and popping out early. Your odds of delivering right on schedule are iffy. A birth two weeks before or after the due date is considered normal.

Q: Can I afford this pregnancy?

Having a child is not fundamentally an "economic" decision, but certainly adding to the family subtracts from the wallet. From a strictly financial point of view, parenthood is a lopsided venture. Imagine a "parenthood ledger sheet." Expenditures: tremendous emotional output and thousands of dollars spent over many years. Income: only love.

But the decision to become a parent comes from the heart, a lopsided organ if there ever was one. There is no "ideal" financial time to have babies, and if people waited for one, maybe there wouldn't be any babies at all. Having a child disrupts normal schedules and budgets, but if it is a welcome disruption, you would not ever wish to return to the stable past. Most parents would agree that a child's love and the parenthood experience are priceless. When there is the will to become a parent, one can find ways to afford it. And there is nothing like a baby to create tremendous economic motivation!

There are as many solutions to the financial impact of parent-hood as there are parents. Early in pregnancy, find out what maternity leave you are entitled to, and whether your partner's employer permits paternity leave. If you anticipate a significant drop in income, you might begin planning for it now. Child-care costs and options vary widely throughout the country. Investigate your area's going rates for in-home child care (live-in and live-out), day-care centers, home-based family day-care programs, etc., so you know what to expect. Though you may feel tempted to "cross that bridge when you come to it," you should keep in mind that in some cities, highly popular day-care programs actu-ally have waiting lists!

Don't be daunted by the high price tags on cribs, strollers, and other paraphernalia. Children do not need top-of-the-line infant swings and designer overalls. Check out discount stores and lower-priced equipment, provided it meets child safety guide-lines. One group of friends passed around a white wicker bassinet for years. It became a cherished tradition for neighborhood new-borns to spend their first few months in that bassinet by the parents' bedside before graduating to a crib.

Welcome relatives' offers of hand-me-down clothes. (Laun-der them before your child wears them.) Your child will create unbelievable mountains of laundry, and it can help to have lots of clothes on hand. Hand-me-downs save you money and enable you to splurge on a few special outfits for dress-up occasions.

Q: Am I too old to have a baby?

Old is not what it used to be. Although an age of thirty-five or older is still considered a high-risk factor, the odds of a normal pregnancy, birth, and baby are excellent for an older mother who is generally healthy and conscientious about prenatal care. A family history of uncomplicated pregnancies boosts your own chances of having one.

Later parenthood may even be an emotional advantage for some. "I needed my twenties and thirties to grow up first," said one woman. "Only then was I ready to help someone else grow up." If being older also means you are more emotionally mature, well established in your relationship and career, and financially stable, then waiting may prove to be a benefit for both you and your child.

However, conceiving may be more difficult if you wait. And older women do have somewhat higher risks of miscarriage, Down syndrome and other chromosomal abnormalities, high blood pressure, heart disease, diabetes, fibroid tumors, deficient fetal nourishment and oxygenation, problems with uterine contractility, and cesarean section. Check with your practitioner to see if you are at particular risk for these conditions. But do not let this somber list dishearten you. Good prenatal care significantly reduces or eliminates the risks.

CHAPTER 2

Taking Care of Yourself and Your Baby-in-Progress

Q: Why are prenatal-care visits important, and what do they consist of?

"I'm not sick, I'm pregnant," said one woman. "So why do I need to see my doctor every month?" She identified the paradox of prenatal care: frequent medical monitoring for a normal physiologic state. But that is the beauty of preventive medicine. It permits earliest detection of any changes from normal health, often before serious symptoms occur. With virtually all medical problems, the earlier they are discovered, the more easily they can be treated.

The goal of prenatal care is to confirm that you and your fetus are healthy and normal, and to help the two of you stay that way.

The First Prenatal Visit

See a doctor or nurse-midwife as soon as you suspect you are pregnant. This may be as early as two weeks after your first missed period, or much later if a history of irregular menstrual periods masks a missed one. The sooner you begin prenatal care, the sooner you can benefit from your practitioner's expert observation and advice. The first prenatal visit includes a complete medical history, examination, certain tests, and discussion of due date and other important matters.

Giving a medical history makes your practitioner aware of any particular problems to watch for. A medical history includes:

- *Menstrual History*
  When was your last menstrual period (LMP)?
  Was it of the usual amount and duration?
  Are your periods regular? How many days usually elapse between periods?
  How old were you when you first got your period?
- *Contraception History*
  Were you using contraception when you got pregnant?
  If so, what type?
- *Pregnancy History*
  How many pregnancies have you had, and what were their outcomes? Include number and dates of live births, abortions, miscarriages, stillbirths, and ectopic pregnancies.
  Of the babies you have had, describe their lengths of gestation (e.g., born at term, early, or late), labor, birth weight, type and place of delivery, condition, and any complications.
  How long did it take you to conceive? Did you need fertility-enhancing medications?
- *Pregnancy Symptoms*
  What are your symptoms (e.g., missed menstrual period, nausea, frequent urination) and when did you first notice them?
- *Medical History*
  Do (or did) you have serious accidents, diseases, or medical conditions? For example, abnormal Pap smear, asthma, blood transfusion(s), diabetes, gynecologic or other surgery, heart disease, hepatitis, high blood pressure, HIV/ AIDS, infertility, kidney or urinary-tract infection, liver

disease, mitral-valve prolapse, neurologic problems including epilepsy, phlebitis, psychiatric problems, rheumatic fever, sexually transmitted diseases (including chlamydia,
genital herpes, gonorrhea, hepatitis B, human papilloma
virus, syphilis, etc.), thyroid dysfunction, tuberculosis, varicosities?
Are you allergic to or have you had any complications with
anesthesia, drugs, or medications?
Are you Rh-sensitized? (See section on Rh Incompatibility
in Chapter 9, "Potential Concerns," page 119.)

- *Substance Use*
Do you smoke?
Do you drink alcohol?
Do you take any illicit drugs, such as marijuana, cocaine,
heroin, amphetamines, barbiturates, etc?
These practices can be harmful to the fetus. Your prac-
titioner can suggest methods or refer you to programs that
can help you stop. (See Chapter 11, "Drugs, Alcohol,
Cigarettes, and Caffeine," page 138.)

- *Genetic Factors*
Are you thirty-five or older?
Do you and/or your partner have other children with, or a
family history of, cystic fibrosis, Down syndrome, hemophilia, Huntington's chorea, mental retardation, muscular
dystrophy, neural-tube defect (such as spina bifida or anen-
cephaly), sickle-cell anemia or sickle-cell trait (most common among black people), Tay-Sachs (most common
among Jewish people), thalassemia (most common among
those of Greek, Italian, Mediterranean, or Oriental descent),
or any other inherited genetic or chromosomal disorder?
Do you have a family history of twins?

Examination. You will be weighed and have your blood pressure taken. These "baseline" figures enable you and your prac-

titioner to calculate net weight gain and blood-pressure changes over the course of your pregnancy.

Your practitioner will give you a pelvic examination to confirm pregnancy and determine how long you have been pregnant (the age of gestation). From the doctor's perspective, a pregnant woman's pelvic exam is distinctive. The cervix is soft and blue or purple. The uterus feels globular and soft where it joins the cervix. The ovary that generated the egg that was fertilized feels enlarged and tense. The pelvic exam is also important for evaluation of your "pelvic architecture," the size and shape of your pelvic bones. This is a reassuring moment for many petite women who erroneously assume that their pelvises will be too small to permit vaginal birth. How one looks on the outside is not necessarily how one is built inside. A woman who wears a size-four dress may have a roomy pelvis, while her size-fourteen friend may not. A key factor, of course, is the baby's size. Here heredity does you a favor, since a smaller woman is more likely to give birth to a smaller (though healthy) baby—especially, of course, if the baby's father is also smaller in stature.

The pelvic exam and information about your last menstrual period should provide enough information to enable your practitioner to give you a due date. If there is still any doubt that you are pregnant, your practitioner may order a quantitative test for hCG, the pregnancy hormone. Or you can have a sonogram— a "portrait" of your uterus as drawn through ultrasound. Ultrasound is analogous to the sonar that helps ships spot objects at sea. Sound waves are projected, come in contact with an object (e.g., uterus, fetus), and bounce back to a receiver. A "sound picture" is created, and measurements of various objects can be obtained quite exactly: for example, the gestational sac in very early pregnancy (the fluid sac inside the uterus in which the fetus develops), the fetal shell, the femur (long bone of the leg), abdomen, the fetal crown-rump length, and, as pregnancy progresses, various features of the fetus up to and including visualization of the chambers of the fetal heart (through Level III sonography).

If you have not had a Pap test (which screens for cervical cancer) within the last year, have one now during the pelvic exam. Your practitioner will also examine your breasts. If you do not know how to do a breast self-exam, ask your practitioner to teach you. During pregnancy, as during nonpregnant times, it is important to examine your breasts every month and report any lumps or irregularities you find.

You will be asked to give urine and blood specimens for various tests (see chart on pages 133–137). Your practitioner will also discuss diet, vitamins, exercise, and any special concerns. This is only the first of many opportunities to discuss how you are feeling, what you can expect to feel, and anything you are concerned about. Throughout your pregnancy, keep a small notebook in your purse so you can keep a list of questions to ask during prenatal visits. The written list not only reminds you of questions it might otherwise be easy to forget; it can also serve as a diary of your pregnancy.

Don't censor yourself. If questions seem a little silly or embarrassing, they are still probably nothing your practitioner has not heard before. This is what you are paying for: your practitioner's expertise and attention. Establishing an ongoing dialogue enables you to find out what you need to know and helps the practitioner serve you better.

ROUTINE PRENATAL SCREENING TESTS

Test	Purpose	When and How Performed/Comments
Blood Typing	Discover blood and Rh type, as well as any antibodies that	First prenatal visit; uses blood drawn from arm. Blood type must

indicate that the fetus has inherited from its father factors that may be incompatible with the mother's blood, causing her body to immunologically "attack" it as a foreign presence.

be known in case you ever need a transfusion; Rh type to determine whether fetus may be Rh-incompatible. If abnormalities are found, blood tests must be repeated during the pregnancy.

Blood Pressure

Discover whether you have such complications as preeclampsia.

Every prenatal visit; done electronically or with cuff and stethoscope.

Complete Blood Count (CBC)

Produces a "portrait" of the blood, including red blood cell count, hemoglobin and hematocrit, to detect anemia; white blood cell count to detect infection; platelets, a factor in the blood-clotting mechanism; mean corpuscular hemoglobin, to see if a normal amount of hemoglobin is in the blood—a function of iron sufficiency; and mean platelet volume (MPV).

Albumin

Discover whether you have toxemia.

Every prenatal visit; uses urine specimen to determine presence of protein.

Glucose	Discover whether you have hyperglycemia or gestational diabetes.	Every prenatal visit; uses urine specimen to determine presence of sugar. A one-hour glucose-tolerance test is recommended. If necessary, a three-hour glucose-tolerance test is performed.
Rubella Titer	Determine whether you are immune to rubella (German measles).	First prenatal visit; uses blood drawn from arm. If you do have sufficient antibodies, you are immune to rubella. If you don't, be sure you avoid exposure to the disease, especially during the first trimester; rubella can cause birth defects. After you have the baby, get immunized against rubella prior to getting pregnant again. After being immunized, wait at least three months before conceiving.
Toxoplasmosis Titer	Discover whether you are infected with toxoplasmosis, a disease transmitted through cat feces and raw meat. Causes mild symptoms in adults,	First prenatal visit, plus any other time you may have been exposed; uses blood drawn from arm. If infection is found, discuss implications for

	but may cause fetal illness or death.	fetus with doctor and genetics counselor.
Gonorrhea Culture	Discover whether you are infected with gonococcus.	First prenatal visit, and any other time you may have been exposed; analyzes vaginal secretions. Treatment of baby at birth will prevent eye infection.
VDRL	Screening for syphilis	First prenatal visit, plus any other time you may have been exposed to syphilis; uses blood drawn from arm. If you do have syphilis, prompt treatment is important.
Hepatitis B	Screening for hepatitis B	First prenatal visit, plus any other time you may have been exposed to hepatitis B; uses blood drawn from arm.

Tests for other sexually transmitted diseases, such as chlamydia, human immunodeficiency virus (HIV), and others, should be performed if you may have been exposed to them.

Subsequent Prenatal Visits

You may be asked to bring a specimen of first morning urine to every prenatal visit. It may feel strange at first, tucking a vial of urine into your purse before you leave home for the day. But the first morning urine is the most concentrated specimen of the day and therefore the one most effectively tested for glucose (a warning sign of hyperglycemia or gestational diabetes) and albumin (which may indicate toxemia).

At each prenatal visit, you will be weighed and have your blood pressure taken. Your practitioner will check the fetus's position and eventually listen for the fetal heartbeat and let you listen, too. It is a thrilling sound, surprisingly fast, like a horse's gallop. You can invite your partner and children to come into the examining room and hear it, too. For many people, it is the first moment that they truly realize that a baby is growing inside.

If your fetus is small-for-date or if you are pregnant with twins, triplets, or more, the heartbeat(s) may be audible later than usual. Be patient—you will get to hear it before too long.

When you are about fourteen weeks pregnant, your practitioner will say, "Let's measure your fundus." You might reply, "My what?" and wonder what part of your anatomy the fundus is and why you never heard of it before. The fundus is the height of your uterus, which becomes quite impressive as pregnancy progresses. As for the fact that you never heard the term before: If this is your first baby, you've never seen your uterus in full action before, and lots of surprises are in store. Every month since you began menstruating, your uterus has made itself known to you through its monthly shedding of the endometrium (the uterine lining) and perhaps some cramping. But pregnancy is the uterus's time of glory. The rich endometrium gets the opportunity to nourish a fetus. Over the nine months, the uterus gets to stretch like a great balloon with a prize inside, thereby qualifying for fundus measuring.

Q: How do the uterus and the fetus change throughout pregnancy?

The First Trimester

First Month

About six days after conception, the ovum (the fertilized egg) implants in the uterine wall. A yolk sac forms, and its long stalk is taken up into the umbilical cord. The amniotic cavity filled with fluid surrounding the embryo enlarges. The embryo's cardiovascular system develops in its first month, and the nervous and intestinal systems begin to form.

Also set into motion is the development of the system that will help nourish and protect the fetus:

- Through the developing *umbilical cord*, the embryo will receive all nourishment and oxygenation. The embryo's waste products will be removed via the umbilical cord.
- By seventeen to twenty-one days after conception, the *placenta*, an entirely new organ, begins to function on the wall of the uterus. Thousands of villi, fingerlike projections in the uterine wall, combine to form the placenta, a cooperative creation of uterine and embryonic tissue. If the villi that comprise the placenta were "unwound" and laid end to end, the villi would make a thirty-mile-long line.

The placenta is an exchange device, the medium through which woman and fetus communicate.

Through the placenta, you send the fetus oxygen and such nutrients as glucose and amino acids, as well as antibodies to infection. By way of the umbilical cord, the fetus excretes carbon dioxide and waste products.

The placenta is also a manufacturer, synthesizing hormones including hCG, hPL, estrogens, and progesterone, as well as important enzymes. The placenta is often called the "afterbirth" because it is delivered after the baby is born. By the end of pregnancy, the placenta weighs one-fifth to one-sixth as much as the baby, and looks like a hefty spongy pancake. It is, in fact, named after a Latin word for cake.

- The fetus floats in *amniotic fluid.* Early in pregnancy, there is little fluid, but by term there is about 1,000 ml. But amniotic fluid is more than a swimming pool; it is a medium of exchange between woman and fetus. The fetus will actually swallow or "drink" from it, swish it into and out of its lungs in breathing motions, and urinate into it.

Second Month   The ovum has evolved into an embryo a little over an inch long. Its heart beats. Its brain has started to develop, making it extra-important for your diet to be rich in protein, calcium, and iron throughout pregnancy. Limb buds appear. Facial

features, fingers, toes, eyelids, and ears
begin to develop.

Third Month　　　　Now the embryo is called the fetus.
About four inches long, its major organ
systems are formed.

Sexual characteristics start to appear.
The fetus urinates; its blood circulates; its
liver functions. It can open fists and
mouth. Eyelashes, nails, and hair form.

The Second Trimester

Fourth Month　　　　Fetal breathing movements are present
(having begun at about thirteen or
fourteen weeks of gestation, or at three-
and-a-half months). The fetus is about six
inches long.

Fifth Month　　　　The fetus may be ten inches long.
The swallowing reflex develops. Fine
downy hair called lanugo is present on
its body.

At about the sixteenth to twentieth
week of pregnancy, you should feel
movement, also called "quickening." If
you have had a baby before, you may feel
it sooner because you will know what to
expect. If you haven't, it may take some
time for you to realize that the fluttery
feeling inside, like the distant stirring of a
butterfly, is in fact the fetus moving
within its watery world. As the fetus grows
and strengthens over the coming months,
its movements will become so much more
pronounced that you may imagine it to be
the world's most precocious acrobat,
kicking through hoops and somersaulting
on trampolines.

Sixth Month

The fetus is now about a foot long and weighs nearly two pounds. It is skinny, since subcutaneous fat has not yet formed. If the fetus is born immaturely now, it would have a chance of staying alive outside the uterus.

The Third Trimester

Seventh Month

Fat begins to be deposited under the fetus's skin. Weight increases to about three pounds. Reflexes are more developed, and the fetus can suck its thumb. If born prematurely, the baby would be viable.

The fetus is now coated with the vernix, a cream-cheese-like substance.

Eighth Month

This is a key month for growth and maturing. The fetus's weight may nearly double from last month's. Though the fetus's lungs are still immature, it would have an excellent chance of survival if born prematurely.

Ninth Month

The fetus's weight increases to approximately six-and-a-half or seven-and-a-half pounds. It is eighteen to twenty inches long. The full-term fetus more fully fills the uterus, so there is less room for acrobatic feats! Any time during this month the fetus can safely be born, although the safest time is within two weeks of the due date.

Q: *What changes can I expect in my body?*

Think of pregnancy as a theater production: The uterus may be the star, but it is supported by a hardworking ensemble. Pregnancy is a systemwide phenomenon that affects your whole body.

See Chapter 9, "Potential Concerns," for a description of the many changes your body will experience.

Every pregnancy is as unique as a fingerprint. It is quite common to hear a woman say, "I was sick as a dog when I was pregnant with Johnny, but I never felt better than when I was pregnant with Jane." During prenatal-care visits, your practitioner should prepare you for changes you will experience, and you should discuss any concerns you may have.

PHYSIOLOGY OF PREGNANCY

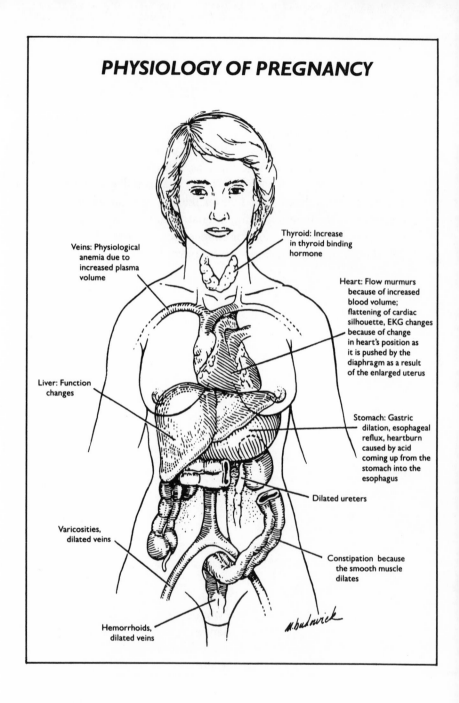

Veins: Physiological anemia due to increased plasma volume

Thyroid: Increase in thyroid binding hormone

Heart: Flow murmurs because of increased blood volume; flattening of cardiac silhouette, EKG changes because of change in heart's position as it is pushed by the diaphragm as a result of the enlarged uterus

Liver: Function changes

Stomach: Gastric dilation, esophageal reflux, heartburn caused by acid coming up from the stomach into the esophagus

Dilated ureters

Varicosities, dilated veins

Constipation because the smooth muscle dilates

Hemorrhoids, dilated veins

CHAPTER 3

Cravings and Cautions: What to Eat and What to Avoid

Q: What do I need to eat or avoid eating?

Eating healthful food can always make you feel good about yourself—and this is especially so during pregnancy. Your fetus eats whatever you do, so you have it within your power to give it a wonderful beginning. Pregnancy can also be an opportunity to learn how to establish healthy habits that will benefit you not only through pregnancy and breast-feeding, but your whole life long.

Eating well during pregnancy is an important responsibility, but it need not feel like a burdensome one. Just as you need to be well rested during pregnancy, you also need to put to rest any of the "food anxiety" to which you may be accustomed. Eating is a "loaded issue" for many women because of our society's obsession with thinness. Women with eating disorders such as anorexia nervosa (literally starving oneself) or bulimia (bingeing and vomiting afterward) reflect extreme, self-endangering reactions to this obsession. But for other women, too, eating is not simply a pleasurable way to fuel the body. It is often an occasion for guilt ("I really shouldn't have this second helping") or strict self-lecturing ("I must have more self-control") or denial ("I am hungry, but if I distract myself, I can hold off from eating"). When you can't have a slice of bread without enduring an inner debate about it, it is time to step back and reorient yourself to a more relaxed approach to eating.

Food anxiety is the last thing you need during pregnancy. By staying within the following guidelines, you can meet both your own nutritional needs and those of the fetus, and relax and enjoy every meal.

Easygoing Eating During Pregnancy

1. *If you eat moderate portions and a healthful, well-balanced diet, you don't need to worry about gaining enough or too much weight.* You will gain what is right for you and your baby. The average weight gain is between twenty and thirty pounds, and reflects:

> 7 to 7½ lb—average baby
> 1 lb—placenta
> 2 lb—increased size of uterus
> 2 lb—amniotic fluid
> 2 lb—increased size of breasts
> 2 to 3½ lb—increased blood volume

An additional five to ten pounds represents helpful fat deposits that serve as "insurance" that you will have the energy and sustenance you need, both during pregnancy and while you are breast-feeding.

While eating well virtually guarantees that you will not gain too much, it is still important to monitor your weight gain. You are in a nine-month marathon; pace yourself accordingly. In the first trimester, gain slowly. As the fetus grows during the second and third trimesters, weight gain will increase commensurately.

Many women manage to increase their weight slowly and

steadily until the ninth month, when they feel so large and sedentary, so "weighed down," that they let their weight soar. Craving extra bowls of double-fudge ice cream probably stems more from emotional anxiety than hunger. Try to get comfort not from food but in other ways: from time spent with loved ones, spiritual readings, rest, warm baths, relaxing strolls. And think ahead: By controlling weight now, you will have an easier time getting your figure back after the baby is born.

But it is not only postpregnancy weight loss that should motivate you. Excessive weight—at any time, and especially during pregnancy—stresses your body. Being overweight taxes your heart, liver, and other organs, and burdens your back, legs, and feet.

For some women, pregnancy is an opportunity to let loose in the kitchen. They figure, "I'm going to gain weight anyway, I might as well have a good time doing it!" They drink milk, but along with it consume an entire box of Girl Scout cookies. They prepare a healthy dinner of chicken, rice, and salad, but have three heaping portions of each. If they do not exercise, weight accumulates especially rapidly. By the end of the third trimester, the "good time" is over, and they are depressed at the prospect of losing all the pounds they've put on.

The bottom line is: For both you and your baby, it is dangerous for you to gain too little or too much.

If you are underweight, you risk fetal malnourishment, intrauterine growth retardation, premature birth, stress, and the depletion of your own body's strength, energy, and overall health.

If you are overweight, it may be more difficult for your practitioner to assess the fetus's development and position and more difficult for you to give birth. You risk excessive fatigue, vascular stress, back and leg pain, and producing a fetus that is too big for vaginal birth. Overweight can be symptomatic of pregnancy-onset diabetes. And overweight people are often as malnourished as those who are underweight, if besides eating too much, they also eat "wrong." Gaining too much weight also presents you with the daunting postpregnancy project of having to shed many excess pounds, just at a time when you will need your stamina and energy to take care of your new baby.

2. *Eat when you are hungry—even if you are "between" meals.* Keep portions small for easier digestion. There is no law that you must eat three large meals a day. In fact, eating smaller amounts more frequently has several advantages. Food is easier to digest. You are likely to eat a greater variety of foods. And you are less likely to eat more than you really want or need, because you will not feel so ravenous.

3. *Make every bite count nutritionally.* Eating whenever you feel like it obviously is most beneficial when what you feel like eating is something good for you. If you primarily eat foods that have a nutritional payoff, you are far less likely to gain excessively. Avoid fried foods and fatty meats. Cutting out refined sugar reduces calories from less nutritious foods, and may improve your overall appearance and mood. So eat, but wisely.

4. *Well, maybe not every bite.* If you are eating nutritious foods, then by all means enjoy a "treat" now and then. Have a dish of ice cream and revel in the knowledge that it is a delectable way to get some calcium. At the same time, consider choosing a treat that may have fewer calories and fat, like ice milk, sherbet, or frozen yogurt, as long as they are not artificially sweetened.

5. *Vary your meals; surprise yourself!* If you are bored with cornflakes every morning, why not start the day with tuna or egg salad on crackers? In fact, since many breakfast cereals are overly refined and sweetened, you may be better off with a high-protein food. Or switch to whole-grain or bran cereals topped with fresh fruit for a light, refreshing lunch.

6. *Do not cheat yourself of the nutrients your body needs.* Your fetus is an unabashed freeloader, driven by the need to grow and survive. It will take the nutrients it needs. So if you do not ingest enough protein, or vitamins, or minerals, the fetus will appropriate those that are available, and your own muscles and

bones and well-being will suffer. You may become exhausted or ill and lack the stamina pregnancy requires.

7. *Avoid overeating by remembering: You are not eating for two; you are eating for one who is pregnant.* The fetus cares that what you eat is nutritious; in terms of quantity, however, it needs relatively little. So don't feel you need to eat twice as much as you want—or that overeating won't matter because you need twice as much food now. Think instead of eating twice as well—but just enough and not more. Your digestive system will thank you. And if you don't gain much over thirty pounds, you will find it easier to regain your figure after the baby is born.

8. *Babies are built of protein—make sure you supply enough.* While high-carbohydrate, low-protein diets are popular for people trying to lose weight, they are not appropriate during pregnancy. When you digest protein, it breaks down into amino acids from which human protein can then be built. There is no question that eating animal protein—meat, poultry, and fish—is the most efficient way to get the protein you and your fetus need. For vegetarians, getting enough protein is a challenge. If you eat fish, eggs, and milk, you will have no problem. Otherwise, you must plan meals carefully to ensure that you are eating enough whole grains, peas and beans, and soy and other high-protein foods. Discuss the situation with your practitioner.

9. *Baby-making takes energy—in the form of calories.* A calorie is a measurement of heat energy, and you need at least three hundred calories more per day during pregnancy to sustain a fetus's growth and development. Obtain calories from carbohydrates and protein (four calories per gram) and fat (nine calories per gram).

10. *Vitamins and minerals are vital.* Each benefits your body in its own way. It is important to know what they do and where to get them. Although vitamin and mineral supplements can be valuable, it is important not to overdose. Do not take *any* supplements unless prescribed by your doctor. Your primary source of vitamins and minerals must be the foods you eat.

Vitamins

Vitamin A builds cells and tissues—bones, teeth, mucous membranes, eyes. Good sources of vitamin A are milk, butter, fortified margarine, cheese, liver, and egg yolk. Carotene, a component of vitamin A, occurs in leafy green and stem vegetables such as spinach, lettuce, asparagus, and broccoli, as well as in carrots.

B vitamins are a complex of various vitamins, including thiamine, riboflavin, niacin, vitamin B_{12}, and folic acid. They aid metabolic (building up and breaking down) changes. Good B-complex vitamin sources are milk, cheese, eggs, leafy green vegetables, yeast, poultry, fish, and whole-grain breads and cereals.

Vitamin C (ascorbic acid) prevents scurvy and perhaps also, to some extent, the common cold. Citrus fruits are vitamin C's best-known sources, but others are strawberries, tomatoes, kale, cantaloupe, cranberries, and broccoli and leafy green vegetables when eaten raw. Vitamin C is destroyed when food is cooked.

Vitamin D regulates the absorption of calcium and phosphorus, aiding the formation of bones and teeth. The best source is sunlight (but never to excess, please); milk with added vitamin D and egg yolk, liver, fish, and fish-liver oils are also fine sources.

Vitamin E may be helpful in reducing fibrocystic breast disease. It is found in whole grains, leafy green vegetables, nuts, dried beans, and animal tissues.

Vitamin K is essential for blood clotting. Get it through leafy green vegetables, cabbage, and cauliflower.

Minerals

Your body and your fetus use minerals to construct tissues and blood. Adequate intake of the vitamin-rich foods listed above also provides the minerals you need. However, iron, and possibly zinc, do need to be supplemented during pregnancy to make absolutely sure that you get enough. Following is an explanation of key minerals, though trace elements of several others, including cobalt and copper, are also important.

Calcium hardens bones and teeth, is a factor in blood and tissue fluids, and aids normal response to nervous stimuli. Recent studies show greater amounts of calcium may be beneficial for pregnant women in some instances. But check with your practitioner before taking calcium supplements, since too much calcium can lead to kidney stones. Ideally, you will get all the calcium you need through your diet, including three to four glasses of milk daily.

Chloride aids acid-base balance and helps maintain osmotic pressure.

Chromium helps the body to metabolize sugar.

Iodine is necessary for proper thyroid function. Using iodized salt protects you from goiter, a disease caused by iodine deficiency.

Iron is crucial to blood formation.

Phosphorus, an element of bones and teeth, helps maintain the blood-buffer system.

Potassium and *sodium* are essential elements of body fluids. Correct potassium balance is necessary for proper cardiac function.

Sulfur helps form healthy skin, hair, and nails.

Zinc helps the body utilize vitamin A and is an essential mineral during pregnancy.

VITAMIN/MINERAL SUPPLEMENTS

Prenatal vitamin and mineral supplements ensure that you get some important nutrients, such as folic acid (vitamin B_{10}), iron, and trace elements such as zinc and chromium that can be quite difficult to get in sufficient amounts through food alone. And when your appetite is low or you feel too stressed to cook, at least you are getting the vitamins you need. There is even some evidence that women who do not take prenatal vitamins may be more likely to have fetuses with nervous-system defects.

But a few cautionary notes are in order:

- Do not exceed the recommended dosage of the prenatal vitamin your practitioner supplies. Fat-soluble vitamins (A, D, E, and K), when taken in excess, accumulate in your body and may be toxic.
- Vitamin C does the opposite; it is excreted daily, so you must replenish it daily.
- Vitamin/mineral supplements are not a *substitute* for healthy eating. It is important, throughout your pregnancy, to eat in sufficient quantity in order to nourish yourself and your fetus, to gain the weight you need, and to supply energy.

11. Movable feasts make eating well easier. The challenge of eating smaller portions of nutritious fare more frequently is to have good food on hand when you are hungry. Otherwise you are at the mercy of the office coffee cart's meager selection and feel so starved that you devour three sugar doughnuts. The trick is to see every storage place as a possible stash for food. That means: Keep melba toast, juice boxes, and cans of peaches in your desk drawer. Claim a corner of the office refrigerator for a little stack of yogurt containers and a carton of milk. Tuck a bag of peanut-butter crackers and an apple in your purse before you leave home in the morning. Store breadsticks, nuts and raisins, and a juice box in your glove compartment. This squirrellike behavior is good practice, by the way, for the movable feasts your child will require, all the zwieback and little bags of Cheerios you will be toting in the future.

At home, make snacking easy by keeping fresh raw vegetables (carrots, cauliflower, celery, green beans) on hand, along with yogurt to dip them in. If you don't want to spend your time slicing and chopping, stock up on crudités at the neighborhood salad bar. Also make six hard-boiled eggs at a time, and tuna salad, and chicken drumsticks, for quick and easy protein.

12. *Don't eat no fat.* That is not an ungrammatical sentence. You *do* need some fat for healthy skin and hair, for processing of fat-soluble vitamins, and for the fetus.

13. *Drink plenty of fluids.* Just as our planet consists more of water than earth, people consist of more water than solid matter. Pregnancy exaggerates the proportions even further, with increased blood volume, and amniotic fluid, and the constant wash of fluids between woman and fetus. Drinking lots of water and juices every day facilitates all this fluid motion. It also aids digestion, helps prevents constipation, helps your kidneys flush out waste products and your urinary tract stay clear of infection, and keeps your skin soft. Water is the best (and no-calorie) drink, but your three to four daily glasses of milk also count. You can also drink fruit and vegetable juices and vegetable broth. Avoid artificially sweetened beverages.

14. *Use salt in moderation only.* The motto "Moderation in all things" certainly applies here. A salt-free diet in pregnancy does *not* protect you from edema (water retention). Edema tends to occur more in women who eat a low-protein, high-fat diet; during pregnancy you need a high-protein diet, along with the small (but necessary) amounts of fat discussed below.

Nor is excessive salt good for you. Avoid salty chips, heavily salted nuts, and sodium-heavy processed meats. Do not use much salt in cooking, either.

Always use iodized salt. If you have problems with high blood pressure, check with your practitioner about your salt intake.

15. *Plan your daily menu around seven food groups:*

LEAFY GREEN AND YELLOW VEGETABLES

Baked squash with a maple syrup glaze, or steamed fresh kale or spinach with a dash of low-sodium soy sauce can add key vitamins and intriguing flavors to your evening meal.

CITRUS FRUITS, TOMATOES, AND RAW CABBAGE

There's always orange juice for breakfast, but have you thought of a midafternoon snack of pink grapefruit wedges? Brighten sandwiches with sliced tomatoes, and try adding shredded raw cabbage to them instead of lettuce.

POTATOES AND OTHER FRUITS AND VEGETABLES

A salad a day will keep your skin glowing, your bowel movements regular, and your eyes sparkling. Pack salads for lunch, or include one every evening for dinner. Salads need not be boring; in fact, they invariably benefit from surprise ingredients, like toasted pine nuts, chopped fresh dill, parsley, or basil, diced apple, raisins or chopped prunes, slices of fennel, celery, raw kohlrabi or turnip. For a protein boost, top salads with cottage cheese, leftover chicken or fish.

Potatoes have acquired an undeserved reputation as a fattening food—it is guilt by association, and nothing more. Yes, potatoes and sour cream or butter have an affinity, but potatoes without the fat are highly nutritious. Bake them and top with yogurt or ratatouille (stewed eggplant, zucchini, tomatoes, and onions) instead of sour cream. Boil tiny new potatoes and add them to soups and salads.

MILK AND CHEESE

Calcium is crucial during pregnancy, and your best way to get it is by drinking three to four glasses of milk every day.

Choose low-fat or skim milk, which provide the calcium you need without the extra calories. Or obtain calcium through other dairy products such as yogurt and cheese.

You need not get bored by glasses of milk and grilled cheese sandwiches. Add nonfat dry milk powder to oatmeal and other hot cereals, to fish chowder, quick breads, and puddings. Blend plain yogurt with fresh fruit; layer it with Grape-Nuts or bran cereal for a quick parfait, or freeze fruited yogurt in ice-pop molds for a refreshing summer snack. Top casseroles with grated cheese; enrich packaged macaroni and cheese by adding some Gruyère or cheddar of your own.

If milk is difficult for you to digest, opt for aged cheeses, cultured yogurt, or milk products labeled lactose-reduced or lactose-free. Remember other sources of calcium, too: fresh steamed greens, canned salmon, or mackerel with bones.

MEAT, FISH, POULTRY, EGGS, PEAS, AND BEANS

Protein builds muscles; make sure your diet is protein-rich. Animal products provide the most efficiently utilized proteins. Dried peas and beans and tofu and other soy products are also good sources for vegetarians and for meat-eaters who seek variety. Try adding tofu to stir-fried vegetables. Stir canned peas and beans into soups, stews, rice, and salads. Mash beans and top with shredded vegetables for a change from the usual sandwich. Eat bean burritos, pack split-pea soup in your thermos (don't forget whole-grain croutons), and enjoy a dollop of yogurt on vegetarian chili made with kidney beans.

WHOLE-GRAIN BREAD AND CEREAL

Shredded wheat, bran, and other whole-grain cereals are a great improvement over highly sweetened processed cereals that masquerade as nutritious breakfasts on supermarket shelves. And a slice of whole-wheat bread offers nutrients that white "enriched" bread can't begin to compete with. For variety, try whole-wheat bread French toast; whole-grain waffles; toasted wheat germ mixed with plain yogurt, sliced banana, and a dash of cinnamon; whole-grain bread pudding; brown rice with raisins.

BUTTER AND FORTIFIED MARGARINE

A couple of tablespoons a day of these, or cooking and salad oils, dressings, or mayonnaise, is all you need. Don't skip them altogether—your fetus's central nervous system contains a significant amount of fat, and you need it, too, for healthy skin, hair, and tissues.

Pregnancy Nutrition Checklist

Every day, make sure you have:

- one or two servings of a citrus fruit or other source of vitamin C
- two servings of other fruits
- one serving of meat, poultry, or fish
- three to four glasses of milk, or the equivalent in the form of yogurt, cheese, or other calcium sources
- three servings of green, leafy vegetables and yellow vegetables
- four to five servings of whole-grain bread or cereal
- two additional servings of any of the above foods
- two servings of fat (one serving equals one tablespoon of butter, cream cheese, oil, salad dressing)
- plenty of water (and fruit and vegetable juices)

Keep track. It may be helpful to keep a list of what you eat, so you will know what you still need and what requirements you have already satisfied. Having the checklist should free you to be able to eat what you are hungry for, when you are hungry for it.

SAMPLE MENU FOR A HEALTHY PREGNANCY

Breakfast:
citrus fruit (orange juice, half a grapefruit)
an egg or whole-grain cereal with skim milk
whole-grain toast or muffin with 1 tablespoon butter
glass of milk

Midmorning Snack:
fresh fruit

Lunch:
salad of fresh vegetables or fresh fruit
chicken, fish, or cottage cheese
glass of milk

Midafternoon Snack:
cheese and whole-grain crackers (preferably those not made with
    hydrogenated oils)
fresh fruit

Dinner:
meat, chicken, fish, seafood, or tofu-bean casserole
two green or yellow vegetables or one vegetable plus a tossed
    salad
whole-grain roll or baked potato or rice or small portion of pasta
fresh fruit

Evening Snack:
hot milk and graham crackers

And remember to drink plenty of water throughout the day.

CHAPTER 4

Exercising During Pregnancy

Q: Shouldn't pregnancy be a time to rest? Why bother to exercise?
When fatigue wraps around you like a soft, heavy shawl, the last thing you feel like doing is taking a twenty-minute walk in the chilly air, driving to the gym for a swim, or even relocating from the couch to the floor for a few stretches. But if you coax your memory to recall past walks, swims, and stretches and the warm, healthy glow you felt afterward, then it becomes easier to shake off the shawl and move.

Rosy cheeks and the virtuous feeling of doing something good for yourself are only two of exercise's many benefits. For pregnant women, regular and reasonable exercise:

- keeps appetite up and weight down
- counteracts sluggish bowels, promotes regularity, and helps prevent or reduce hemorrhoids
- helps prevent insomnia
- provides an emotional lift and helps banish moodiness
- strengthens muscles that support your skeletal structure, so you keep posture straight and avoid backache
- improves breathing
- encourages you to drink adequate amounts of water
- increases stamina and the attitude of positive persistence you will need throughout pregnancy, labor (especially the

second stage, when you need to push the baby out), and motherhood

- improves your ability to keep your balance, especially important later in pregnancy when the heavy uterus can tip you over if you aren't careful!
- improves pelvic musculature

THE DO'S AND DON'TS OF EXERCISE DURING PREGNANCY

DO have fun! Exercise is, or should be, one of life's great pleasures. When you choose activities you enjoy, you are more likely to do them more often and reap greater benefit.

DO s-t-r-e-t-c-h. A gentle series of stretches is a great way to start or end the day, or provide a transition between workday and home time. Always do stretches before aerobic exercise to prevent muscle injury.

DO get your heart and lungs pumping with moderate aerobic exercise:

Walk. A daily twenty-minute walk is the easiest form of aerobic exercise for most women to build into their busy schedules. Consider walking older children to school instead

DON'T regard exercise as bitter medicine you have to swallow. If you tend to live a sedentary life, pregnancy can be just the motivation you need to incorporate exercise into your life. It is never too late to begin exercising, or to surprise yourself with just how good it feels.

DON'T exercise flat on your back. If you do, your uterus presses on the great blood vessels and restricts blood flow to the placenta and fetus. When you exercise on the floor, lie on one side.

DON'T push yourself to exhaustion. Please—moderation in all things, including exercise.

DON'T start off with a five-mile hike. Build distance and time gradually.

of driving them. Get off the bus two stops in advance of your destination and walk the rest of the way. Map out an errand route for a purposeful stroll. Drive to a park with a friend and explore the (not too steep) paths.

Swim. A buoyant experience in more ways than one: especially during the third trimester, it is lovely to feel so light.

DON'T swim alone, or in a crowded pool where you could get kicked or pushed, or in a dirty pool. Do not dive or jump into the pool. Do not swim if you have started to dilate, or if membranes have ruptured, or if your practitioner advised you to stop.

Jog—but *only* if you jogged regularly before you became pregnant.

DON'T start jogging during pregnancy, because you are more prone to injury.

DO Enroll in a prenatal exercise class. You'll feel more secure doing exercises designed for the pregnant woman and enjoy the camaraderie of your classmates. Also explore prenatal yoga classes, or study with a yoga teacher whom you can trust to tell you which exercises (such as inverted postures or those that overstrain abdominal muscles) to avoid.

DON'T take regular exercise or dance classes unless you know which exercises to avoid. If classes are rigorous, they may exhaust or strain you.

DO Consult your practitioner about such activities as skiing, skating, tennis, golf, biking, and horseback riding. The determining factors are the strenuousness of the activity, the

DON'T begin any of these activities during pregnancy. If your practitioner gives you the go-ahead to continue activities, monitor your energy and stop when you are tired. Don't ski on

level of your skill, and your ability to resist injury and maintain your balance.

high mountains, where the high altitude could deprive you and the fetus of oxygen.

DON'T participate in any contact sports such as touch football, or in other activities that could cause injury, such as scuba diving, mountain climbing, skydiving, or waterskiing.

DON'T use exercise machines that could strain your muscles, or vibrating machines that could stimulate premature contractions.

DON'T use saunas, hot tubs, or otherwise expose yourself to high heat.

ADAGIO: REFRESHING STRETCHES TO DO AT HOME

Many ballets begin with fast, energetic music, then segue into adagio, when the music slows and the dancers slow their motion, taking forever to extend their legs into space. For many dancers, this is the heart of the dance: no rush, just the sensation of stretch.

As a busy pregnant woman, find time for adagio in your life. The following exercises, some of them yoga stretches, fulfill a double purpose: to tone muscles and to help you relax. The exercises follow a progression from top to toe and incorporate breathing techniques that will assist you during labor. Consciously inhaling and exhaling through the movements will enhance your experience and help keep motions even.

Create an oasis of beautiful music and let each exercise fluidly lead to the next. Before long your muscles will remember the movements on their own, and you may want to improvise beyond them.

BEFORE YOU BEGIN:

1. Wear loose, comfortable clothing.

2. Take your phone off the hook or turn on the answering machine so you can exercise undisturbed.

3. Do not eat for the hour preceding exercise.

4. Empty your bladder.

Equipment:

Place an *exercise mat (or blanket or quilt)* on the floor. Have ready a *sturdy chair* for support during standing exercises, and *two pillows* for use during one of the breathing exercises.

PHASE ONE: FLOOR EXERCISES

Put on slow, rhythmic music that you love, that moves you to move. Sit on the exercise mat, legs folded in a comfortable tailor-seat position, knees out and feet tucked underneath. (Fig. 1)

Begin with Calm Breathing.

- **Cleansing Breaths.** With hands loosely resting on your lap, close your eyes and relax with "cleansing breaths," inhaling through your nose for three counts, and exhaling through your mouth for three. Repeat five times.

Relax Your Face.

- **Tighten and Release.** For three counts, tighten your face muscles, squeezing eyes and mouth shut, then release into calm. Repeat three times.

- **The Lion.** (Fig. 2) Now reverse the process to open the face. Kneel and sit back between your heels. (If this is difficult, stay in the tailor-seat position.) Place hands on

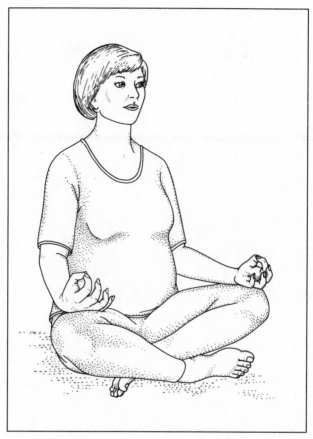

Fig. 1

your knees. Inhale and spread your fingers like a lion about to spring—but lift only slightly off your heels and keep hands on your knees. At the same time, open your mouth in a silent leonine roar, stick out your tongue as far as it can go, and gaze upward. Hold the inhalation for a count of ten, then release and exhale. Repeat the exercise three times. This exercise tones facial, neck, and hand muscles.

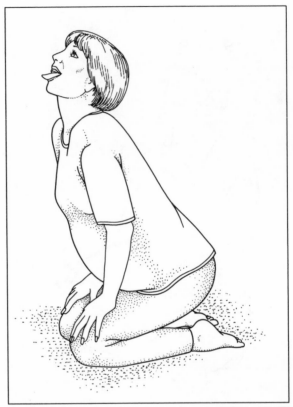

Fig. 2

Release Tension from Your Neck.

- **Slow Head Rotations.** Either kneeling or sitting tailor seat, with back straight, close your eyes and lower your chin to your chest. Inhale and very slowly roll your head to the right shoulder and to the back, then exhale as you complete the rotation to the left shoulder and forward again. Keep the movement smooth and relaxed. Do two head rotations to the right and two to the left. The neck is a repository of tension for many people; do this exercise several times during the day to relax neck muscles.

- **Follow the Gaze.** Continue in the sitting position, back straight but relaxed. Keeping your face forward, let your eyes gaze to the right as far as they can, then inhale and slowly let your face turn to the right also, as though you are trying to look over your shoulder. Gaze left and exhale, letting your face follow the gaze back to center. Keep your movement smooth, never jerky. Repeat to the left side. Repeat exercise two times. This exercises your eyes and neck.

Relax and Tone Your Upper Body.

- **Slow Shoulder Rotations.** Sitting with a straight, relaxed back, inhale, and smoothly rotate shoulders forward as far as you can, then up to your ears, and exhale for the continued rotation back and down. Repeat four times, then rotate shoulders in the reverse direction five times, inhaling for the rotations back and up, exhaling as shoulders roll forward and down. Shoulder rotations can relieve upper-back tension any time during the day.

- **Breast Toning.** With elbows bent, press palms together in a prayer position. Inhale, hold for five counts, then exhale and release pressure. Repeat five times. (Fig. 3)

  Then stretch elbows back so that hands part (Fig. 4); return briefly to the original position (Fig. 5), then straighten arms outward as you again extend arms back. (Fig. 6) Keep back straight so that lower back does not indent. Repeat five times.

- **Rib Cage Shift.** Continue to sit straight. Inhale and gently shift rib cage to the right, and exhale as you return to center. Repeat to the left.

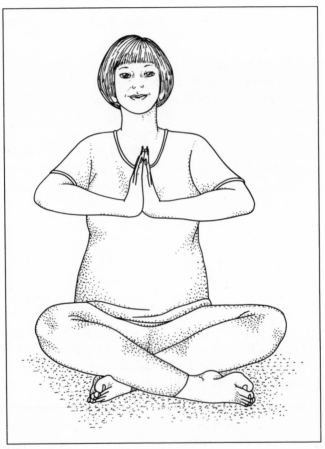

Fig. 3

Open Your Back and Pelvis.

- **Spine Flexibility.** (Fig. 7) Sit with knees bent, feet touching. Grasp ankles. Inhale, then as you exhale gently lower your head and round your back. Inhale as you gently straighten from the base of the spine up, so that you straighten your back before you raise your head.

- **Hip/Groin Stretch.** Keeping your left leg bent, with your left hand holding your left ankle, extend your right

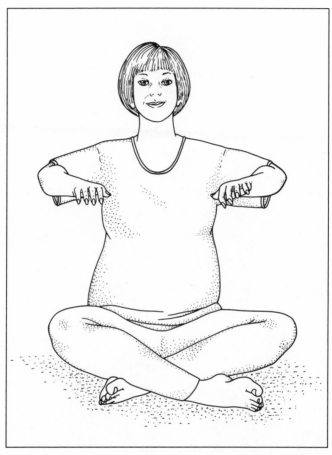

Fig. 4

leg along the floor. Inhale as you simultaneously press your left foot close to your groin and flex your right foot. Hold for ten counts, exhale, and reverse direction. Do the exercise three times on each side.

- **Pelvic Stretch.** (Fig. 8) On your hands and knees, exhale for a slow count of three as you round your back, keeping head down, then inhale for three counts as you straighten your back and raise your head. Repeat five times.

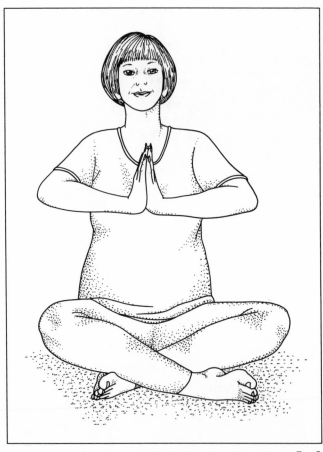

Fig. 5

Improve Foot and Calf Circulation.

- **Foot Rotations.** Extend both legs in front of you and lean back on your hands for support. Slowly rotate your right foot five times to the right and five times to the left. As with previous rotation exercises, inhale for half of each rotation and exhale as you complete the rotation. Repeat with the left foot.

- **Foot Flexes.** Continue to extend both legs in front of

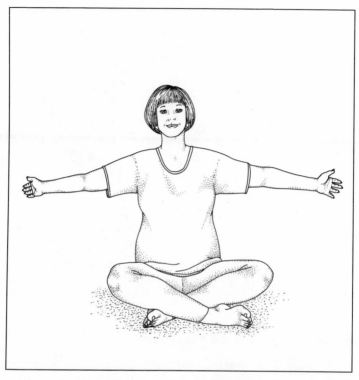

Fig. 6

you and lean back on your hands for support. Inhale and gently push heels forward so that feet flex and toes point to the ceiling. Exhale and reverse so that feet point forward gently (not in an exaggerated balletic *pointe*). Repeat ten times.

- **Foot Massage.** Leaning your back against a wall or a solid piece of furniture for support, keep your right leg extended, bend in your left foot, and gently massage your left foot, including each toe, the full sole and ankle, and your calf. Repeat with the right foot.

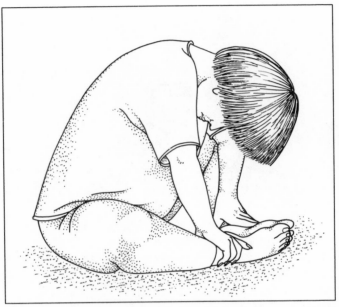

Fig. 7

Breathing Exercises to Aid You During Labor.

- **Complete Breath.** Sitting in a comfortable position, back still supported, breathe in through your nose as deeply as possible, feeling the air fill your lungs. Slowly exhale by letting air hiss out through your mouth. This breathing technique is especially helpful during the first stage of labor, when contractions last for thirty to forty seconds each.

- **Slow Chest Breathing.** Take a Complete Breath (described above), follow it with six to nine shallow throat breaths, and conclude with another Complete Breath. This technique is valuable when contractions are stronger and last longer.

- **Panting.** With mouth open, pant with short, shallow breaths, as a dog does on a hot day. Use panting breaths

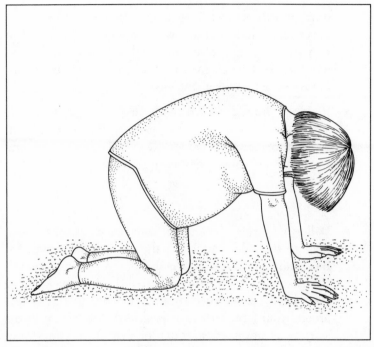

Fig. 8

during the pushing stage of labor when your practitioner asks you to stop pushing.

PHASE TWO: STANDING EXERCISES

Rise slowly to standing. If necessary, hold on to a chair for support so you do not lose your balance. Check music to make sure you continue to have its company. Have a sturdy chair ready for support.

Lengthening Stretches Move Upward and Outward.

- **Sideways Stretch.** Assume a comfortably wide stance, with legs about two feet apart. Keeping your back straight, inhale and raise your right arm overhead, stretching upward as though trying to touch the ceiling with your fingertips. Exhale and follow the stretch to the left, your right arm touching your ear. Inhale to rise to center and repeat to the left. Do exercise five times in each direction, always keeping movement fluid.

- **Picking Grapes.** With both arms overhead, gently stretch one arm up, then the other, as though you are in an arbor reaching for grapes. Keep breathing smooth and steady. Stretch ten times with each arm.

Toning Arms.

- **Ballerina Arms.** Standing with back straight, open arms to the side, parallel to the floor, palms down. Inhale and raise arms on a count of five, slowly rotating palms toward each other, until fingertips touch above your head, your arms forming an oval picture frame around your face. Exhale as you slowly lower arms to the starting position on a count of five. The slower your count, the more you will benefit from the exercise. Repeat five times.

- **Arm Circles.** With arms straight out at your sides, parallel to the floor, palms down, rotate arms in very small circles ten times, then in the reverse direction for ten times, keeping arms straight. Then have palms face the ceiling and do two more sets of arm circles, one in each direction.

- **Wrist and Finger Limbering.** With arms straight in front of you and hands in loose fists, rotate wrists ten times in one direction and ten times in the other. Then open your fingers like the petals of a flower, and close them like a bud, letting them do their own adagio dance to the music.

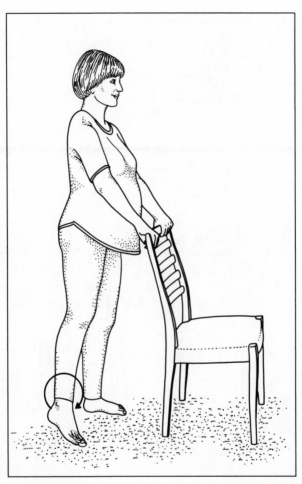

Fig. 9

Limbering the Hip Sockets.

- **Leg Circles.** (Fig. 9) Face the back of the chair and place both hands on it for support. Stretching the right leg straight, trace low circles in the air with your toes, five times in one direction and five times in the other. Repeat with left leg.

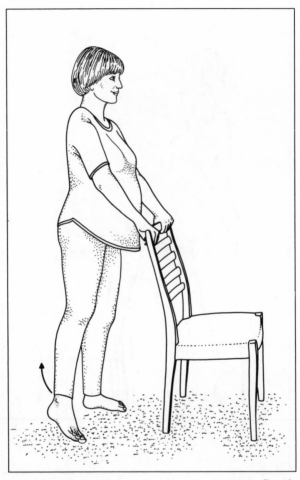

Fig. 10

- **Leg Lifts.** Continue to use the chair for support as described above. Lift left leg to the side (Fig. 10), then return foot to center and do a shallow knee-bend with feet together. (Fig. 11) Repeat with right leg. Do five leg lifts with each leg.

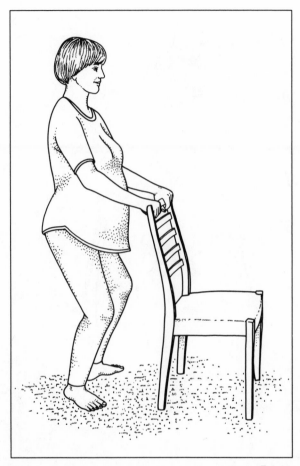

Fig. 11

- **Calf Stretches.** (Fig. 12) Still holding the back of the chair, extend your left leg back, foot touching the floor, and press your heel to the floor ten times. Repeat with right leg.

PHASE THREE: COOLING DOWN

Centering Breaths. Stand still, eyes closed. As you inhale, let arms float up to shoulder level, then exhale and let arms float

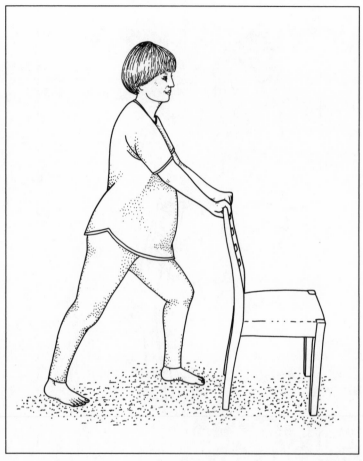

Fig. 12

down, doing a slight knee-bend at the close of the movement.
Repeat three times. Then simply stand still for another few moments, preparing to make the transition from your adagio oasis.
Try to carry your relaxed, calm feeling through the rest of the
day. Open your eyes, and smile.

CHAPTER 5

"I'm Not Fat, I'm Pregnant!"

Q. How will I feel as my shape changes through pregnancy?

At first, probably unreal. Intellectually, you know you are pregnant. You may *feel* pregnant (tender breasts, morning sickness). And yet when your pregnancy begins to show, you may very deliberately have to coach yourself not to think of these changes as "fat," but as the outward evidence of the life growing within you. Women are so accustomed to wincing when they widen that pregnancy requires almost a shift of vision. If you, like many women, are in the habit of harshly scrutinizing yourself for signs of overweight, now is the time to learn a new way of seeing. A simple, even amusing visualization trick can help you get used to getting bigger: As if you were gifted with Superman-type "X-ray vision," imagine that you can "see" the fetus growing within you when you look at yourself in the mirror. It is a lovely image, one body nested within the other, like a Russian Matrioshka doll. Especially use this image any time you might feel tempted to skimp on food so you will not look "fat." Keep your mind clear, and your body—and your fetus—nourished.

You may feel more comfortable with your body when your pregnancy is more obvious, because at that point there is no confusion: These are the contours of pregnancy, not the turnoffs of flab.

But expect to have good days and bad days, due to pregnancy

hormones' erratic mood effects and your own process of adjustment. At times, you feel flushed with pride, graceful as a blossom, buxom, and highly sexual. On less rhapsodic days, you long simply to tie your shoes without a world globe in the way, and to ride your bike without concern about keeling over. And you look forward to once again being able to decide whether to shop in a certain store on the basis of its merchandise, not the wideness of its aisles.

Carrying a watermelon-size uterus certainly changes space perception. One pregnant woman, invited to a Christmas party at her new boss's home, wondered why her hosts had designed their kitchen with so little space between the counter and work island, where the buffet was set up. She found it difficult to load her plate and maneuver over to her space at the table. But at the following year's Christmas party, months after her baby was born, she realized that in fact there was ample space in the kitchen—now that *she* was smaller!

Q. When should I start wearing maternity clothes, and how should I choose them?

Maternity clothes are what women buy when not even a long rubber band looped through a buttonhole can keep their favorite skirt closed anymore. It is one of the milestones of pregnancy: that first expedition to the department store to buy maternity clothes. You'll notice, as you wend your way down the aisle, that just outside the maternity department is a display of sweet, tiny layette items for newborns: frilly pink doll-size dresses and cozy yellow sleepers. But stay focused; time enough later to indulge in buying baby clothes. Right now, take care of you.

Sometimes women put off buying maternity clothes because they pride themselves on staying somewhat svelte thus far: the triumph of good abdominal muscles from years at the gym. Or they've waited because they have not announced their pregnancy yet and fear that maternity clothes will nonverbally but surely announce that a baby is on the way. That will be the case especially if you choose pink gingham empire-waist frocks, or one of those proud-mama T-shirts that sport a big arrow pointing to the abdomen with the words "Under Construction." At some point, however, perhaps around the fourth month, earlier if this is not your first pregnancy, you will simply not find your regular clothes wearable. And though a roomy caftan or your husband's big shirt worn over a pair of leggings may serve you well, you still need clothes that will see you through the coming months in style and comfort. Even the most generously cut dresses will not work for long, because your pregnant belly will cause them to ride up in front. Maternity clothes are cut to accommodate your growing size.

It can be one of the great treats of pregnancy to select clothes that you really love. This is a time to buy fewer things and maybe spend a little more on clothes whose colors, fabrics, and style give you a lift. For weekends, buy a pair of jeans, a couple of pretty shirts, and a big, cozy sweater. For work, buy tops and bottoms that mix and match, and a blazer or two to tie them together. To get you from season to season, layer lighter fabrics, like cotton, rayon, and fine wool, instead of investing in heavy winter clothes that you may not wear often. Jumpsuits are fun, but not if they have a million buttons that will annoy you every time you have to go to the bathroom. If you expect dress-up occasions, you might want to invest in a season-spanning dress, or just get a fancy top, pair it with pants or a skirt, and complete the outfit with jewelry. You may also have friends who can lend you maternity clothes, which is especially helpful for costly items like jackets, suits, and evening wear.

Don't sneer at maternity panty hose; they really are more comfortable, and regular ones will not stretch enough. You probably do not need maternity underpants, however, since regular cotton bikini underpants are likely to be cheaper and just as comfortable. But definitely buy one or two bras that give your breasts adequate support.

Some women try to be superpractical and buy clothes they

expect to wear after pregnancy, too. Certainly, postpartum it will take time for your uterus to contract to its normal size and for you to lose any excess pounds, so you will be wearing maternity clothes beyond your baby's birth day. But once you no longer look pregnant, you are unlikely to want to wear maternity clothes; you will want to move on.

And now a word about the need to buy larger clothes for a *nonpregnant* person: your spouse. It is by no means a scientifically documented fact, but many people believe that a number of men gain weight when their pregnant wives do. They give new meaning to the phrase "pregnant couple."

At first your partner may think the clothes dryer is overzealous, suddenly shrinking his favorite T-shirts. But belts don't shrink. When your man progressively fastens his belt one, then two, then three notches away from the usual well-worn spot, it is a telltale sign with which he cannot argue: He's rounding out just like you. He may even feel sympathetic aches and pains. Not to worry, though: He can join you in exercise and healthy salads to keep weight gain to a minimum. And postpartum, the couple who gained weight together can lose it together, too.

CHAPTER 6

The Pregnant Couple

Q. How will my partner feel about my changing body?

The August 1991 issue of *Vanity Fair* magazine challenged readers throughout the country to consider just how they felt about a pregnant woman's changing body. The magazine featured seminude photos of the actress Demi Moore, eight months pregnant. Readers' responses ranged from delight and admiration to outrage and disgust. The latter reaction was an interesting throwback to the days when pregnant women had to take their walks at night, so no one would see their altered form. People are used to seeing naked women on scores of magazines at the local newsstand, but those women's sexuality has not, at least according to the photos, progressed into maternity. But a pregnant woman visibly attests to having had sex; she has blossomed from it. To many people, there is no more exquisite sight than a pregnant woman's body; they see the ripening of life.

You may be apprehensive over your partner seeing a rounder you. Yet your partner may be more attracted to you than ever, stirred by the beauty that the two of you created together, and proud that he has fathered a child. And he may even feel more uninhibited sexually, knowing he does not have to think about birth control!

Enjoy pregnancy; connect with your own sexuality, and your partner will, too. Some women, in fact, feel their sexiest and most voluptuous when pregnant. Their breasts are bigger, their round belly is a feminine and earthy sight. One woman even said it was a relief having a round belly: She didn't have to worry about whether her stomach looked flat! If pregnancy is cause for celebration, then your being visibly pregnant is a celebratory sight, a sign of the bond you and your partner share.

Q. *How can I involve my partner more in the pregnancy?*

Ask him to join you occasionally at prenatal-care visits. Listening to you ask questions of your doctor or midwife will encourage him to ask his own questions. He will be thrilled to hear the fetal heartbeat and gratified each time he hears the words "Everything's normal. Looking good!" If you have a sonogram, the sight of the fetus will help pregnancy seem more real for both of you—and provide the first picture for your baby book.

Shop together for maternity clothes, nursery furniture and wallpaper, the layette. Have fun going through baby name books. How many couples have collapsed in laughter—"Does anyone really *name* their baby that?"—and adopted some droll nicknames for the fetus that sometimes even became nicknames after birth. Initiate conversations about how life will change when the baby is born, about your fantasies and dreams.

Let him help you. One woman felt embarrassed by how often she vomited during her pregnancy, until she realized that her husband felt good about taking care of her and ministering to her needs. Pouring the glass of seltzer, buying the saltines, wiping her face with a wet washcloth, and stroking her hair gave him the opportunity to express his love, to share somehow in the physical stress she alone had to endure.

Use these months before the baby comes to have special times together. Take off for a weekend trip and stay at a bed-and-breakfast inn. Go for walks together, pack a picnic, meet for lunch. Sleep in together on Sunday mornings and spend the afternoon in bed, too, reading the paper, making love, and feeling the baby move. One man's favorite memory of his wife's

pregnancy was of hanging out together on lazy Sunday after-
noons. He liked placing his hand on her naked stomach and
feeling the fetus roll around. At first, he felt only twitches or
waves. But in the third trimester he'd watch in amazement and
make them both laugh by calling a play-by-play like a sports
announcer: "I think that's a knee! There—that's definitely a fist
poking out."

Attending childbirth classes together has become almost a
standard pregnancy ritual and can bring couples closer. The
classes not only teach your partner how he can help you when
you are in labor, they also give him the opportunity to observe
other men with their partners, and to share pregnancy tales.
Many couples have formed lasting friendships with other members of their childbirth classes.

Q. *How will my relationship with my partner change?*
The poet Walt Whitman wrote in *Leaves of Grass* of the
"year that trembled and reel'd beneath me!" Pregnancy might be
compared to that sense of upheaval. It is months of constant
change that test the stability of the love that created it.

Pregnancy tends to magnify, not transform, the quality of a
relationship. It may increase intimacy for an already close couple,
and exacerbate the conflicts of a couple whose relationship has
been "trembling and reeling" for a long time. Certainly, pregnancy cannot be counted on to be a solution to a rocky marriage.

However, pregnancy can provide a context for renewing your
connection with your partner. The more time you spend together, the more involved your partner is, and the more you
make decisions jointly, the better prepared you will be to carry
the spirit of cooperation and kinship into parenthood—when, if
anything, the tests of a relationship are even greater.

Q. *Is it okay to have sex during pregnancy?*
Sex has been called the glue that holds marriages together.
Pregnancy is an important time to enhance togetherness, and

sex is one important way to do it. Unless your practitioner cautions you against making love during pregnancy because of specific miscarriage risk or complications, sex can be a rewarding and exciting part of your pregnancy.

Pregnant women are not by nature fragile; they are not eggshells about to crack. Yet for eons the myth that pregnant women should not have sex was alive and well. In fact, some pregnant women feel their sexiest during pregnancy. Freed of the need for birth control, of the idea that they should look skinny and flat-stomached, and of any anxiety about whether they *could* get pregnant, many women find sexual relations with their partners exceptionally satisfying. Some even find it easier to attain orgasm during pregnancy.

In the first trimester, nausea and fatigue may cancel out sexual desire, and in the third trimester a couple must call forth extra ingenuity to figure out how to connect comfortably. However, several other factors can inhibit a couple's sexual activity:

- *"We are not alone."* Objectively, you realize the fetus doesn't "see" you in bed, or "know" you are having sex. But the feeling of a third presence may interfere with your pleasure. Think ahead to when the baby is born and starts to cry the minute you two start to kiss. Now *that* is a third presence, and a demanding one!

  Remember that it was the act of love that created the fetus in the first place; sex keeps renewing the love that will make your family a nourishing one for the baby.
- *Fear of harming the fetus.* Yes, the fetus is small and fragile, but it benefits from the best packaging nature has to offer. The fluid-filled uterus protects its small inhabitant, and the cervix is a tightly closed door shielded by the mucus plug. A top-security setup, if ever there was one.
- *Fear of inducing labor.* For most of pregnancy, sexual arousal is unlikely to cause labor to begin. Ask for your

practitioner's advice, however, about having sex in the last month or so of pregnancy.

Do not have sexual relations if your partner has or suspects he may have a sexually transmitted disease (STD).

- *Self-consciousness about your changing shape.* How sexually close a couple is depends largely upon their willingness to be vulnerable, exposed, and open with one another—not only physically, but verbally, too. If you feel unsure about whether your pregnant body is still attractive, confide in your partner. Chances are he still finds you sexy, but perhaps he did not realize that you needed reassurance.

- *Awkwardness.* As you grow bigger, you and your partner can experiment with alternative sexual positions. Lying on your back will become too uncomfortable, but lying on your side or being on top eliminate any pressure on your uterus and give you more space and control. The important thing is to connect sexually, and intercourse is not the only way to do that. Kissing, stroking, massage, mutual masturbation, and oral sex can all be satisfying alternatives. The only caveat: When your partner performs oral sex on you, make sure he knows never to blow into your vagina. This could cause a fatal embolism in your bloodstream.

CHAPTER 7

Ups and Downs

Q. *I was so thrilled to be pregnant, I thought I'd spend the whole nine months in the clouds. So why do I feel so blue?*

Pregnancy hormones cannot account for all of your ups and downs. Pregnancy is an intense time of adjustment, transformation, and preparation for a major life change. *Of course* you might feel seized by anxiety. You might awaken in the middle of the night with an intense feeling of claustrophobia: "This pregnancy is continuing, I cannot get out of this—I have made a commitment to change my whole life, and suddenly I am not sure that's what I want." At one time, these were unspeakable thoughts, akin to jinxes and taboos. Shouldn't you feel grateful to be pregnant? Shouldn't you shut out misgivings and give yourself over to the miracle of creating new life? Ads portray glowing pregnant women, dreamily drinking milk. Yet here you are, pacing the floor in the middle of the night, racked with doubt. What's wrong with you?

You are normal.

For too long, the normalcy of such feelings was not discussed. They were "pregnantly incorrect." But greater openness about how pregnancy—like virtually every aspect of life—is a mixed bag of emotions, has freed many women to talk about their real feelings.

There is a great release when you feel able to express not only hopes but also fears, to mention not only joy but also sleepless nights. Being able to be yourself—your own complicated self— will enable you to cope much more easily with pregnancy, and then motherhood. No mother is always the clichéd smiling woman bearing a tray of home-baked cookies. No pregnant woman need feel that she must always be the tranquil bearer of the next generation.

It is important to have people with whom you can speak openly about what you are going through. Your partner, of course, who probably has his own concerns about becoming a father. Your mother, sister, close friends. And there is nothing like sharing aches and pains and recipes and tips and thoughts and ideas and jokes with other pregnant women. If you do not have any friends who are pregnant at the moment, make some. Strike up a conversation in the dressing room before or after prenatal exercise class, or ask your practitioner to recommend a pregnancy support group.

Two women who worked for the same organization got pregnant only weeks apart. Being able to count on one another for emotional support throughout their pregnancies made all the difference. They compared notes on how they were feeling, shopped for maternity clothes, enrolled in a lunchtime exercise class. One day, one of the women was feeling especially blue. She had just found out that her fetus was in a breech position that would make a cesarean necessary, and she'd had her heart set on natural childbirth. They skipped exercise class and went instead to a coffee shop to talk over a couple of milkshakes. But both women were so large by now that they could not fit into any of the booths or even sit at the counter. They burst out laughing, the humor of their shared predicament making them both feel better.

CHAPTER 8

Pregnant and Employed

Q. Will pregnancy affect my ability to do my job?

Many if not most employed women continue working during their pregnancies and maintain their level of performance. But that does not mean that nothing has changed. Most women find it unrealistic to try keeping up their prepregnancy pace; something has to give. Referring to her smaller store of energy, one woman said, "I give at the office. When I come home, I collapse. After dinner I get right into bed. I talk on the phone or read, and I'm asleep by nine o'clock." Her co-workers view her as a dynamo; only her family knows that she is able to maintain her energy at work by "vegging out" at home.

Of course, that is harder to do if she has other children, who simply cannot understand why Mommy can't go bike-riding with them instead of napping on the couch. Ideally, her husband or a baby-sitter can take the children out instead. But when such relief is not at hand, even young children can often be bargained with: "I'm too tired to take you out bike-riding now, but while I rest on the couch, I'll mend your Batman doll's cape." Or read a story, watch a video, be an appreciative (and sedentary) audience for their puppet show. If you absolutely cannot keep your eyes open another minute, children old enough to safely play on their own for twenty or thirty minutes might better accept your boring need for sleep if you set a timer or alarm clock and promise to awaken when it goes off. That trick helps them control their impulse to awaken you, since they need not fear that you will nod off indefinitely.

A great way to relax is by relaxing your housekeeping standards. One woman took comfort in her grandmother's wise words, "Don't worry about dust. It will always be there tomorrow." In other words: Put yourself first, not your broom. A pregnant working woman should try not to aim for the Employee-of-the-Year Award and the Good Housekeeping Award at the same time. (Advice that also applies to working mothers.)

Your workaday habits may need to change in response to your needs as a pregnant woman—and the changes may be surprisingly positive and productive:

- Sitting still for long periods of time is uncomfortable now. So for the first time, you begin to build in some breaks— and notice that standing up and walking around a bit refreshes you for a new bout with the pencil when you return to your desk.
- If you commute by bus or subway and cannot get a seat at rush hour, you might negotiate an earlier or later starting time (and corresponding quitting time) with your boss— and discover that the new schedule suits you and your job better than before. Arriving earlier at work may make the most of your "morning person" energy; arriving later is good for "night owls" who like to sleep in.
- Your new need for a noontime walk or nap invigorates you and results in a more productive afternoon.
- If you shift from a full- to part-time work schedule, you may, like many women, discover that you accomplish almost as much as you did before, because you are more focused and better rested from your days off.
- You may have to endure some good-natured kidding about your more frequent snacking ("Baby's hungry again, huh?") but your pregnancy may evoke a gentle helpfulness

from co-workers that is very touching. Colleagues who observe your changing form may even take on a proud, almost proprietary attitude. The attitude brings out a family feeling in the workplace that can be lovely—and from which your child will benefit. Many women, for years after their baby is born, find that their children can't wait to go to the office with them because other employees coddle them so.

There is one small problem you might face. Co-workers who are fascinated with your pregnancy may reach out to stroke your stomach—as though it were no longer a part of you. Some women do not mind this, but if you do, simply say, "I'm not comfortable with that," or "I'm ticklish, please don't."

- At times you find yourself distracted by pregnancy. Your need to urinate more frequently breaks up your day—but consider it nature's way of making sure you get up often enough from your desk! At times, the distraction has a more profound meaning: During a meeting, you feel the fetus move inside you, and the secret sensation is so delicious, you feel flooded with love. At such moments, your perspective changes: Work is important, yes, but your identity as a woman, as a creator of new life, has its own power and beauty independent of anything in the workplace. Anxiety over a late memo or deadline pressure softens a bit in comparison with the pleasure your baby-to-be gives you with its playful, capriciously timed jig.

Q. *I work at a computer. Will this harm my child?*

Recent studies indicate that working at video display terminals (VDTs) is not known to increase your risk of miscarriage or birth defects. However, long hours spent working at a computer may be stressful for *you.* Try to take an hourly break. Stretch, walk around a bit, do head and shoulder and ankle rolls to release tension. An ergonomically designed chair with arms can help support your elbows and spine. Or position a pillow behind your back to help your posture.

Q. *Are there other workplace conditions I should be concerned about?*

Certain chemicals and substances can be hazardous to pregnant women. Anesthetic gases and lead are two that have been documented, but a number of others are believed to be reproductive hazards as well. Ask your employer for information, or contact the National Institute for Occupational Safety and Health's toll-free technical information number (1-800-356-4674) about chemicals specific to your workplace. In general, avoid exposure to substances you are not sure of. For example, if insects or mice in your home or workplace need to be exterminated, do not apply pesticides yourself, and arrange to be absent when they are used.

Q. *How long can I continue to work?*

At some point during pregnancy, nearly all pregnant women hear of their counterparts in bygone days or faraway places who toil in the fields throughout pregnancy. As the tall tale tells it, these superwomen labor in the fields virtually through labor, returning to work shortly after giving birth with the infant strapped to their back. Such superheroism reflects a harsh, impoverished life, and should not be construed as a model of the stoic ideal.

Yet some women pride themselves on not allowing pregnancy to affect their work lives in any way. They become contemporary stoics, the modern-woman version of the woman in the fields. Denying or disavowing stress may help some women cope with demanding work and personal lives. But repressing awareness of stress could backfire for others. Stoicism is not the "right" way to be pregnant; there is no "right" way, except to be aware and attentive to your own needs and those of your fetus and family. A woman who *does* experience the stress of pregnancy is not deficient; she has not failed by being inadequately stoic/heroic.

She should not require herself to be as a goddess, immune to common human travails.

Consult your practitioner about what is the healthiest work schedule for you. Take into consideration your state of health and energy level, as well as the financial impact of the decision. It is certainly possible for some women to work right up to the day they deliver and to return to work speedily. But do try to take advantage of maternity leave to which you are entitled, or try to find a way you can afford to take some time off.

CHAPTER 9

Potential Concerns

Q. *What potential complications should I know about?*

Here, in alphabetical order, are some special concerns and conditions associated with pregnancy. Some are commonly experienced; a few more serious complications are less common but important to know about.

Back Pain. During pregnancy, your pelvic bones loosen in preparation for childbirth. The relaxed pelvic structure places extra stress on the spine to compensate. At the same time, the increased weight of your uterus pulls you forward. Lower-back pain may result. There are several ways to prevent or reduce back pain:

- *Move like a dancer*, never letting your spine collapse into a question mark. A dancer stretches tall and uses abdominal and buttock muscles to keep her lower back flat rather than curved. Though of course your beautiful, round pregnant belly precludes you from having a dancer's willowy silhouette, you can still strengthen these muscles with the exercises described in this book.
- *Modify your daily actions* to minimize risk of back pain. Move long and vertically throughout the day. When lifting something from the floor, do not bend over from the waist, which can strain your back. Instead, stand with

feet wide enough apart to give you a stable base, keep your back straight, and bend your knees to lower yourself. Grasp the package (or child, or bag of dog food), press feet down, and rise straight to standing.

- *Sleep on your side* to relieve pressure on the circulatory system. Support your belly with pillows or rolled-up blankets, and place a pillow between your knees. Recline like a royal sultana surrounded by cushions and ottomans. Use a firm mattress or place a bedboard between mattress and box spring.
- *Wear low-heeled shoes.* Leave both high heels and ballet slippers in your closet. Opt for shoes that give you a little lift with wide, low (not flat) heels.
- *Get off your feet.* Rest your feet on the coffee table or on some of those omnipresent throw cushions with which you surround yourself these days.
- *Relieve backache with warm compresses or gently warm baths—never hot ones.* Be careful getting in and out of the tub.

Breech. Children do not always cooperate with their mothers, and neither do fetuses. By about the eighth month, they are supposed to lie head-down within the uterus, poised for birth. Breech is what happens when the fetus presents buttocks first:

- *frank breech*—sitting with legs flexed at the hips, extended at the knees, buttocks facing the cervix, as though to be born mooning;
- *complete breech*—breech presenting, but limbs fully flexed at both hips and knees;
- *single footling breech*—one foot leading
- *double footling breech*—both feet leading

Breech is detected both through ultrasonography and, commonly, when the practitioner palpates (feels) your uterus through a systematic laying on of hands called Leopold's maneuvers, as well as by vaginal examination.

Breech can be exasperating but does not always require cesarean section. Some breech fetuses turn on their own prior to labor. Some doctors manually turn the fetus, often with the aid of ultrasound. Manual turning, also called "version," should only be attempted by practitioners highly experienced in the technique, because of potential danger to the fetus from the manipulation or a loosened placenta. Skilled practitioners can also undertake vaginal delivery of a baby in frank or complete breech position, provided that: the baby is neither too large nor premature and small; the maternal pelvis is adequate; the fetal head is adequately flexed; the labor is satisfactory; and skilled personnel are present who are practiced in vaginally delivering breech babies. Cesarean section is the safest method of delivery for other breech positions.

Breech presentation during one pregnancy is not a predictor of breech in subsequent pregnancies.

Another alternative fetal position, though not a breech, is the **transverse lie,** when the fetus lies horizontally across the uterus. If the fetus does not turn, safe vaginal delivery is impossible, and a cesarean section must be performed.

Breast Changes. Breast swelling and tenderness or pain are one of the first signs of pregnancy. Breasts may begin to enlarge as early as seven to ten days after ovulation. As pregnancy progresses, the areola, the pigmented area around the nipple, darkens and increases in size, and tiny glands called Montgomery follicles appear. You may notice stretch marks, called *striae*, on your breasts, but they are caused less by actual stretching than by hormonal changes. Also normal is swelling of breast tissue, sometimes under the armpit. If you are worried about any swelling, consult a doctor.

Sometimes the nipples secrete fluid, which in some women appears spontaneously after the first few months of pregnancy.

Some call the fluid *colostrum*, while others reserve that term for the liquid the newborn baby drinks from its mother's breasts immediately after birth (a drink rich in antibodies that confer passive immunity to the newborn).

You might wish to be fitted for a bra by an experienced department-store or lingerie-shop clerk. She can check bras to make sure they give you the support you need. In the third trimester, you may want to buy nursing bras you can use when the baby is born.

You can prepare for breast-feeding while you are pregnant. Keep nipples soft and pliable with lanolin cream or cocoa butter. Do not use alcohol or soap, especially during the last trimester or while breast-feeding, because they can remove the nipples' natural protective oils.

Gently massage your nipples with a slightly twisting motion to get them used to being handled. If you have flat or inverted nipples (if in doubt, ask your practitioner), you can encourage nipples to protrude for easier breast-feeding by using special breast shields. The shields provide a mild suction, which draws nipples out enough so that the baby will be able to fit its mouth over them and suck.

Some breast-feeding counselors also recommend cutting small holes in the tips of your bras so that the friction of nipples against the fabric of your clothing gently desensitizes nipples. You can accomplish the same goal by buying nursing bras that have a flap that lowers and leaving the flap down sometimes so your breasts are exposed within your clothing. Exposing nipples to open air is also helpful—try sleeping naked or relaxing naked or seminude at home.

Cardiovascular System Changes. During pregnancy, your heart works 30 to 40 percent harder because it must pump a higher volume of blood. Pregnant women have 50 to 60 percent more blood than nonpregnant women, because blood carries nutrients to the fetus and transports its wastes.

Yet a harder-working heart is not necessarily a strained one. Just as the menstrual cycle indicates that pregnancy-support systems are in place (that your body "expects" and prepares for pregnancy), your heart, too, is designed to be able to accommodate the higher blood volume pregnancy brings. Pregnancy is not your usual state, but it is still a normal one. At the same time, regular monitoring is important to ensure that all is proceeding normally.

- *Blood pressure.* Blood pressure normally falls slightly during pregnancy. Increased blood pressure is a hallmark of the hypertensive disorders of pregnancy, including pre-eclampsia and eclampsia (formerly called toxemia). These disorders cause blood pressure to climb, tissues to swell, and protein to leak out of the kidneys and pass in the urine; in their most serious state they can lead to convulsions and coma for the woman, and severe risk to the fetus. Smokers are especially at risk of high blood pressure. Because smoking constricts blood vessels, blood must push harder to pass through them.

    Your urine is checked for protein at each prenatal visit to permit early detection of these disorders. Early symptoms include swelling of the feet and excessive weight gain; later symptoms include swelling of hands or face, headaches, dizziness, and seeing spots before the eyes. At the end of the second trimester or in the third trimester, nausea, vomiting, and abdominal pain may also indicate these disorders, and may even indicate an emergency situation.

    The key thing to remember is: *If hypertensive disorders are caught early, they are easily treated; if allowed to progress, they cause life-threatening situations.* Be alert to symptoms and report any to your practitioner without delay.

    Many women have "war stories" of bouts with such disorders over which they triumphed; in subsequent pregnancies, such women took special care to follow their doctor's advice to get enough rest, to follow a proper diet, to get checked regularly for protein in their urine, and to monitor weight gain, blood pressure, and any development of edema.

- *Ruling out anemia.* Although you have more blood in your body during pregnancy, the amount of blood plasma increases faster than the number of red blood cells. Blood composition must be checked regularly to detect any anemia as soon as possible. Anemia occurs when there is not enough hemoglobin in the blood to transport the oxygen needed by both woman and fetus. Hemoglobin is the oxygen-carrying molecule in red blood cells. Since the body uses iron to manufacture hemoglobin, the most common form of anemia during pregnancy is iron-deficiency anemia. You can prevent and treat it by taking iron supplements and by eating iron-rich foods every day, such as meat, liver, green leafy vegetables (spinach, kale), peas and beans, dried apricots, prunes, raisins, and whole-grain bread and cereal.

  However, neither you nor your practitioner should automatically take it for granted that iron deficiency is the cause of anemia in your case. There are many types of anemia. To name just a few: Pernicious anemia is caused by a deficiency of vitamin B_{12}; folic-acid anemia by a deficiency of folic acid, a B vitamin. Sickle-cell anemia, a serious illness, is an inherited disorder that primarily affects blacks. Red blood cells malfunction when they become misshapen, assuming the shape of sickles. Blood should be tested to confirm which type of anemia you have so the proper treatment can be prescribed.

- *Mitral-valve prolapse.* The most common heart condition in pregnant women is mitral-valve prolapse, also known as a floppy mitral valve. Mitral-valve proplapse can be confirmed through a painless test, echocardiography, which uses sound waves much as sonography does. The condition is benign, but it does pose a small hazard of heart infection during delivery, because bacteria are released that circulate through the bloodstream and can settle in the heart valve, causing subacute bacterial endocarditis. Therefore, depending on the extent of the mitral-valve prolapse, your cardiologist may prescribe prophylactic antibiotics for you to take during labor and delivery.

- *Arteriosclerotic heart disease.* This disease narrows blood vessels and forces the heart to work extra hard, especially during pregnancy. Eating a low-cholesterol diet reduces your risks of getting arteriosclerosis.
- *Diseased heart valves (not including mitral-valve prolapse).* If you have diseased heart valves, whether from childhood rheumatic fever, congenital heart disease, or other causes, the stress of labor can overload the heart. Teamwork among you, your practitioner, and a cardiologist can help you carry the pregnancy to term at reduced risk. Your doctors can prescribe drugs that increase the heart's efficiency; bed rest will further help you avert heart failure. Severe valve disease may rule out your going through the exertion of the pushing stage of labor. The baby can be gently delivered by vacuum extraction or by outlet forceps application. Both methods are described later in this book.

Constipation, Gas, and Hemorrhoids. Pregnancy-related hormones cause sluggishness in the intestinal tract, and pressure from the weight of the uterus can slow elimination still further. Constipation and gas may result. If constipation causes you to push too hard during bowel movements, you may get hemorrhoids—distended anal and rectal veins that can itch or cause pain or bleeding. They may also be hormonally related. If you are bleeding, do not take it for granted that it is from hemorrhoids; consult a doctor.

Following are ways to prevent constipation—both to prevent hemorrhoids and relieve any you already have.

- *Exercise.* Get your system moving. Walking every day for twenty minutes to an hour counteracts that sluggish colon. Also do the exercises that are described in this book.
- *Drink plenty of water every day.* This will help create softer stool that is easier to pass. Fruit and vegetable juices, especially prune juice, are also beneficial. But remember that water contains no calories and is beneficial to your entire system. Do not drink caffeinated beverages that can irritate your colon (besides not being healthy for the fetus), or carbonated beverages that can cause gas.
- *Include fiber in your diet:* whole grains, bran, and raw or lightly steamed fresh vegetables and fruits. If you are unaccustomed to such foods, you may find that they cause gas and discomfort. Add them to your diet gradually and in small portions until your body gets used to them.
- *Don't rush.* Allow time for a bowel movement after breakfast and dinner. If it doesn't happen easily, do not push. Try again later. Heed the urge to move your bowels rather than postponing bowel movements for a more convenient time. If you respect your body's signals, they will serve you well and help you establish regularity.
- *Do "buttock press" exercises* every day. Tightening and relaxing anal sphincter muscles tones them and increases circulation.
- *Relieve pressure on hemorrhoidal veins* by sleeping on your side and not standing for prolonged periods of time.
- *If stool is hard to pass, apply petroleum jelly to the anus.* Heavily advertised hemorrhoid medications are often little more than high-priced lubricants. Regular use of petroleum jelly is a gentle, effective, and inexpensive way to soothe the anal area.

If you *do* get hemorrhoids, do not use any medication, creams, suppositories, or other substance without first checking with your practitioner. Do not take any mineral oil by mouth, or any medication that is not prescribed by a physician. Take warm sitz baths to relieve hemorrhoidal discomfort.

Contractions. Well in advance of labor, usually starting in the second trimester, you will experience your first uterine contractions. Your belly becomes hard and taut as a basketball, and the sensation may stop you in your tracks. But in a minute or so, the contraction subsides as easily as surf recedes from the shore.

You may be surprised to experience contractions at this stage of pregnancy; you probably were not expecting them until labor began at the end of your ninth month. But pregnancy is a continuum, and labor contractions are just the same as those that occur earlier in pregnancy. In labor, of course, contractions are longer, stronger, closer together, and accompanied by cervical effacement and dilatation, and birth. But the uterus essentially performs the same tensing/release action in every contraction, no matter when it occurs.

For years, contractions prior to the onset of labor were nicknamed "Braxton-Hicks contractions," as though they were phenomena distinct from "regular" (i.e., labor-related) contractions. This "distinction without a difference" is dangerous, for it leads some women to dismiss contractions as "nothing," when in fact they sometimes are a sign of premature labor. *Any contractions, any time during pregnancy, may indicate labor and should be reported to your practitioner.*

Cramps. Occasional cramping during pregnancy is very common, caused by the contracting of uterine muscle. You may also feel cramping after orgasm, since sexual arousal can result in uterine contractions. Such cramps do not hurt the fetus and should not alarm you. However, do notify your practitioner of painful or persistent cramps, especially if they occur in your lower abdomen (whether on one side only or in the center). They may indicate ectopic pregnancy or miscarriage in early pregnancy, or a tendency to premature labor later on.

Diabetes. If you are diabetic, and especially if you became diabetic as a child or teenager ("juvenile diabetes"), yours is a "high-risk" pregnancy, and prenatal care is particularly important.

Diabetes sometimes begins during pregnancy. "Gestational diabetes" lasts only as long as the pregnancy, and you return to normal after birth, but if it is not properly treated, the condition can be dangerous to the fetus.

If you are a "borderline" diabetic, i.e., predisposed to the disease, the stress of pregnancy may tip your insulin balance enough that you become diabetic and remain so for the rest of your life. Glucose-tolerance tests to rule out diabetes are important for all pregnant women. At special risk of developing diabetes during pregnancy are women who:

- have a family history of diabetes
- are obese or gain excessive weight during pregnancy
- have a history of two or more miscarriages, stillbirths, or fetal malnutrition
- have delivered babies who had especially low or high birth weights
- have had preeclampsia (toxemia) or polyhydramnios (too much amniotic fluid) in previous pregnancies or currently

Complications for the Diabetic

Prior to the introduction of insulin therapy, there were fewer diabetic pregnant women because juvenile diabetics either did not live into their childbearing years or were sterile. Adult-onset diabetes usually did not appear until after the childbearing years.

Insulin therapy has enabled diabetics to live active, fulfilled, and longer lives. But the complications of pregnancy for the diabetic woman remain, and can be life-threatening for woman and fetus if not closely monitored.

For the woman, sugar tolerance may decrease in reaction to the placenta's production of a hormonelike growth substance called placental lactogen. The nausea and vomiting that are so common during early pregnancy may cause acidosis (when the blood's pH level is below normal). Pregnancy may also bring about retinopathy (deleterious changes in the retina of the eye), nephropathy (deleterious kidney changes), nephritis (kidney disease), hypoglycemia (low blood sugar), ketosis (presence in the urine of ketones, substances that indicate that diabetes is out of control), and possibly puerperal (postpartum) infection signaling the need for changes in insulin requirements.

The fetus of a diabetic woman is at risk of becoming too large, unable to be delivered vaginally; such babies, who weigh over nine pounds, are called *macrosomic.* The fetus of a diabetic woman also has a higher risk of stillbirth because of compromised circulation to the fetus, a greater incidence of hypertensive disorders of pregnancy, and the altered glucose metabolism. The apparently normal-weight or overweight newborn may have immature lungs and respiratory distress, because it is actually premature, though overweight. Hypoglycemia is noted after birth, as the fetal pancreas, used to processing abnormal levels of glucose, overproduces insulin. Congenital anomalies are also more frequent. If the woman has cardiovascular complications, the fetus may not get enough oxygen and other nutrients and be born underweight and malnourished, or be stillborn.

Good News for Diabetic Women

By adhering to the following six-step plan, you can greatly reduce your risks of complications for yourself and your baby. This plan has enabled many diabetic women to produce healthy children and remain complication-free themselves.

1. *Select an experienced obstetrician, and begin prenatal care as early in pregnancy as possible.* Diabetes translates into "high-risk pregnancy," and a doctor rather than a nurse-midwife is better able to give you the care you need. Your best bet is a doctor affiliated with a large teaching hospital that has a neonatal intensive-care unit in case complications occur. If you develop diabetes after you have already begun prenatal care with a nurse-midwife, switch to a physician or request consultation with the physician with whom your nurse-midwife is affiliated.

2. *Eat a high-protein diet, and make sure that you take in enough calories.* Diet is always important during pregnancy; for the diabetic woman it can be the single most critical factor in determining your pregnancy's outcome. Your diet should be individually tailored for you by your obstetrician working in collaboration with a nutrition expert.

3. *Get plenty of rest but also sufficient exercise.* Counteract the stress of pregnancy by going to bed early, resting periodically during the day, and paring down your schedule to prevent burnout.

4. *Avail yourself of a range of monitoring techniques to detect any problems early.* These include glucose monitoring by your doctor and yourself, regularly at home as prescribed (using a glucose meter), ultrasonography, nonstress tests, biophysical profiles later in pregnancy, and amniocentesis. During labor it is important to monitor uterine contractions, fetal heart rate, often fetal blood pH, and to know the fetal position, presentation, and size, as well as cervical dilatation and the descent of the fetus through the birth canal.

5. *Participate in a support group with other pregnant diabetic women.* Both pregnancy and diabetes can provoke anxiety. A support group can help you cope with this "double whammy."

Some pregnant diabetic women have what one researcher called "feelings of defectiveness and shame," along with guilt at having a condition that potentially endangers the fetus. Any dietary lapses or complications can compound such feelings and cause stress that can worsen their condition. Complicating the picture even further is the resentment some women feel toward parents from whom they inherited the disease. A support group helps banish bleak feelings. It reassures you that you are not alone and enhances your ability to stick to your dietary regimen and prenatal monitoring. No support group available? Ask your doctor to help you start one.

6. *Agree to early delivery if tests indicate fetus is overlarge or placenta is deteriorating.* Inducing labor or scheduling a cesarean section can be lifesaving for your baby in such instances.

Edema. Swelling of the feet and legs due to water retention is quite common during pregnancy, especially on warm days. Though bothersome, it is usually nothing to worry about, but let your practitioner know and evaluate the situation.

Wearing support stockings, putting your feet up or resting on your left side, and trying not to stand or sit too long can alleviate the swelling. Keep circulation moving by taking a ten-to twenty-minute walk every several hours. Wear comfortable shoes that do not squeeze your feet.

You might think that this show of excess fluid means you should not add to it. The reverse is true. Drinking plenty of water every day helps the kidneys flush excess water out of your system.

Edema is not usually a reason to totally ban salt from your diet. But neither should you give salt a free rein. Avoid very salty foods like chips, pretzels, and sodium-processed meats.

Persistent, severe edema is a symptom of preeclampsia. Early symptoms are swelling of the feet and sudden weight gain; later symptoms include swelling of hands or face, headache, dizziness or spots before your eyes, nausea, vomiting, or abdominal pain.

If you have one or more of these symptoms, or if edema of the feet lasts beyond twenty-four hours, notify your practitioner at once.

Endometriosis is a condition rarely seen in societies where women have children early. But in our society, where childbearing is often delayed, it is a common problem in women in their late twenties and thirties who have not yet had children. Deposits of womb lining (the endometrium) are found in the abdominal cavity in various locations, most commonly behind the uterus on the ligaments, but sometimes on the bowel or on organs such as the ovaries, causing cysts. The deposits cause scarring. Infertility can be a result of endometriosis. The condition can be treated through drugs or surgery. But interestingly, if a woman is able to become pregnant, that may be the best "treatment" of all, since it causes the endometriotic deposits to regress and the condition to improve.

Fatigue. "Why do I feel so tired?" many pregnant women ask, as if they should be able to sustain their usual energy level. Sometimes fatigue during pregnancy feels like a magic cloak suddenly thrown over you, an irresistible desire for sleep to which you feel compelled to succumb at once. It is not the drained feeling of exhaustion that occurs at the end of a long day, or because of stress or illness. This quieter lassitude announces: Your energy is needed internally now. Obeying that inner command, if only for a fifteen-minute rest, can leave you refreshed and revitalized.

When you sleep, blood is redirected from the muscles that do active work, and the blood supply to the uterus is increased. The fetus gets more oxygen and other nutrients. So sleeping benefits both you and your fetus, almost as though you each "work" alternating shifts.

Don't try to be a hero and struggle on with your normal schedule. Do not ignore fatigue; add naps to your schedule. Getting enough rest will enable you to accomplish more, feel more in control of things, and enjoy a happier state of mind. Naps cushion you from getting worn down and help you ward off illnesses.

At work, if you have your own office, declare time-out for fifteen minutes, close the door, put your feet up on the desk, and close your eyes. Some companies have facilities where employees can nap during lunchtime or on breaks. One woman, lacking such space, sometimes spent lunchtime eating and then resting in her car. Consider taking a bus instead of driving home so you can rest while you commute. Naturally, that applies only if you are sure of getting a seat! When you are visibly pregnant, getting a seat on a bus can be easier. Chivalry is not dead.

If you are home with small children, nap when they do. If they do not nap, insist on a "quiet time" when they play by themselves on their beds (or on yours) while you sleep. Or ask your husband to take charge while you nap.

Retire earlier at night and set your alarm for a bit later in the morning. See if you can shorten your workday. A note to your employer from your doctor explaining your need for rest may be helpful.

Sometimes fatigue may be a signal that you need nourishment. Drink orange juice or eat a piece of fruit. Carry nutritious snacks with you so you can respond right away to flagging energy.

Fibroids are benign uterine tumors. They tend to occur more frequently in women over thirty and can occasionally impede conception or provoke miscarriage or preterm labor. Most women, however, are able to conceive and carry to term even if the fetus must share the womb with fibroids.

Pregnancy hormones may spur fibroids to enlarge, often to the point where they outstrip their own blood supply and degenerate. In such cases fibroids can cause pain and may necessitate a brief hospitalization, but seldom must they be removed surgically during pregnancy.

Fibroids can interfere with efficient contraction of the uterus after the baby's birth, and thus may be a cause of excessive bleeding, or postpartum hemorrhage. However, this is an atypical scenario; most women with fibroids have no such postpartum complications.

Groin Pain can occur when round ligaments attached to the uterus stretch as the uterus enlarges. These "growing pains" are especially common during the third trimester.

Hair Changes. During pregnancy, your hair is more oily, and you may need to wash it more frequently. Your hair also appears fuller and thicker because hormonal changes keep old hairs from falling out at their usual rate. Your new mane is temporary, however. Several months after you give birth and hormones return to normal, the old hair will begin falling out, and you may be appalled at the clump that blocks the bathtub drain. Do not worry about it; you won't go bald. But do alert your hairdresser to what is happening and adjust your style to the lessened volume. Consult a doctor if hair loss seems extreme.

Headaches and Dizziness. Mild headaches, common during pregnancy, may be caused by tension. Interpret them as a signal that it is time to rest. Lie down with a cool washcloth on your forehead, and the headache will vanish in time. If necessary, take an acetaminophen tablet. But never take aspirin. It can impede fetal development and, if taken during the third trimester, complicate labor and delivery. Aspirin interferes with the hormone prostaglandin—a vital ingredient for successful labor. Aspirin can also prevent blood from clotting, which can cause you to hemorrhage.

Occasional dizziness may also indicate a need for rest. You might also feel dizzy if you stand up suddenly after lying down. Sit for a minute first, then slowly rise to standing.

Headaches or dizziness may also happen when you are hungry.

Eating *before* you become hungry will keep your blood sugar at an even level.

Always report fainting, frequent or severe headaches, and recurrent dizziness to your practitioner, who should check to make sure you do not have preeclampsia, high blood pressure, or other medical problems.

Heartburn refers to the burning sensation in the esophagus at about heart level that is caused by backed-up stomach acid. Pressure from your growing uterus crowds your stomach and pushes acid back more frequently.

Eat smaller, more frequent meals. Take small bites and chew thoroughly so that food is better digested once it reaches the stomach. Spicy, fatty, and greasy foods worsen heartburn, so opt for blander fare. Wear comfortable clothing that does not bind your midsection and increase pressure on your stomach. At night, sleep with two pillows under your head so acid flows down, not toward your mouth.

If these measures do not work, ask your practitioner to recommend a low-sodium antacid that is safe during pregnancy.

Hormonal Changes. Pregnancy hormones are the reason pregnancy feels like no other time. They are why your moods sometimes lighten or darken for no discernible reason, why you are nauseous, why your nipples may leak colostrum, why labor begins when it does and not earlier or later. Although some hormones' functions are well known, others are still mysterious. What is known for sure is that somehow each hormone knows what to do, and knows when to bow out when pregnancy (or breastfeeding) ends.

The pregnant body is a hormone factory. Some hormones you produce yourself, others are manufactured by the fetus and placenta. Starting at conception and winding down at birth, you produce at least six protein hormones and a number of steroid hormones, including progesterone, androgens, and more than twenty different estrogens.

Each hormone has its own special tasks. Some hormones can be isolated from your urine, blood, or amniotic fluid and analyzed to determine whether they are present in sufficient quantity. Too much or too little of any given hormone alerts the practitioner to be on the lookout for certain problems.

Some hormones aid fetal development, while others work to prepare breasts for lactation. Among hormones' roles are increasing your oxygen consumption, basal body temperature, frequency of urination, and body-fat stores. Hormones also decrease your energy level and slow intestinal transit time. Pregnancy hormones are like instruments in a symphony: Each has its score to follow and does not necessarily play in unison with the others. Some hormones, like hCG, are the first sounds heard, while others, like oxytocin, which peaks in labor, chime in more toward the end.

A look at hCG (human chorionic gonadotropin) demonstrates how versatile hormones can be. HCG had its Warholesque fifteen minutes of fame in the mid-seventies when hCG was coveted as a diet aid. Pregnant women's urine became like fool's gold, mined for the hCG it contained. Trendy clinics charged hundreds of dollars for hCG injections. But it turned out there was no magic elixir: HCG does *not* burn fat away. If only it did, think of what a lucrative sideline you might have over the next nine months!

Today hCG is prized instead as one of the most reliable clues to whether a woman is pregnant, and to how the pregnancy progresses. Its presence in urine announces pregnancy. Too little hCG in urine can mean impending miscarriage or ectopic pregnancy, a dangerous condition in which the fertilized egg begins to mature in the Fallopian tube instead of the uterus. Too much hCG can indicate the presence of trophoblastic tumors (hydatidiform mole and choriocarcinoma that are tumors of placental tissue).

Like other pregnancy hormones, hCG plays multiple roles. First, hCG stimulates the corpus luteum, a structure in the ovary formed after the release of the egg, to increase progesterone production and support the embryo's growth for the first eight or nine weeks, until the placenta is established. Second, if your fetus is male, hCG helps its testes form. Third, hCG is believed to be immunoprotective. That means that it convinces your body to embrace the fertilized egg, not reject it as a foreign substance. Finally, hCG stimulates the formation of the fetal adrenal cortex. (The adrenal gland is an endocrine gland that sits atop the kidney.)

Hypotonic Uterine Contractions describes inadequate dilatation of the cervix and descent of the fetus due to inefficient uterine contractions. If all else is normal, then pitocin can be judiciously administered by infusion pump to enhance contracting.

Immunology of Pregnancy. It doesn't make sense. Organ transplants—of hearts, kidneys, lungs—often fail because the recipient's body, obtusely unable to distinguish helpful from harmful foreign matter, rejects them. So then why doesn't a woman's body reject a fetus, half of whose genetic material is from its father? Early researchers, stymied in their attempts to figure out this contradiction, concluded only that the uterus is simply "a privileged site," or a "unique milieu." Others have identified the roles of certain substances, such as hCG and EPF ("early pregnancy factor"), in staving off rejection. One theory holds that miscarriage, stillbirth, and placental malfunction may occur because the woman's immunologic system works only too well— rejecting, as with transplants, foreign matter the woman would wish her body to welcome.

Another theory posits that birth occurs because, after nine months, the woman's body no longer tolerates the presence of foreign matter. A stunning coincidence occurs: The woman rejects the fetus just when the fetus is capable of surviving outside her.

Incompetent Cervix. A cervix's job is to keep the entrance to the birth canal tightly closed until pregnancy has come to term. Sometimes, however, a cervix proves unable to stay shut under the weight of the growing uterus; it opens painlessly (without labor), often in the fourth or fifth month, sometimes causing a second-trimester miscarriage. A pregnancy can often be saved, however, by stitching the cervix shut until a time closer to the due date. This is often done under general anesthesia.

Insomnia. One night in your third trimester, you may lie awake wishing that you could fall asleep as easily now as you did in your first trimester. Then, you could nap at the drop of a hat. Now, it is often hard to get comfortable. Or you have to go to the bathroom. Or you simply have a lot on your mind. You mentally flip through a Rolodex of potential baby names. You worry. You make mental lists of things to do and try to resist turning on the light to write them down. You turn onto your left side, then onto your right. You'd give anything for a good night's sleep, but you won't take anything for one.

Except hot milk. Once in a while, it helps. So does exercising before bedtime, which can tire you just enough to lull you into sleep. A warm bath or a gentle massage may also do the trick. If your mind is churning, record your thoughts in a pregnancy journal. Once the thoughts are on paper, you no longer need to be their custodian; you can go to sleep.

Insomnia does have a silver lining: It gets you used to interrupted sleep—which is what you will have when the baby is born.

Kidney Changes. Your kidneys work harder during pregnancy. They must process much more liquid than usual because of increased blood volume and the fetus's output. Kidneys operate more efficiently if you drink plenty of water.

Though most women's kidneys are perfectly capable of functioning well during pregnancy, women with preexisting kidney disease are more prone to pyelonephritis, an infection of the kidneys. Pregnancy hormones cause the ureters, the tubes leading from the kidneys to the bladder, to relax and widen. Urine may form a stagnant pool, where bacteria may cause infection. Premature labor may result. Treatment involves hospitalization, bed rest, and prescription of antibiotics that will not harm the fetus.

Another possible problem is kidney stones. They are painful to pass at any time, and especially upsetting during pregnancy. Before the advent of ultrasound, kidney stones were difficult to diagnose because most practitioners try to avoid kidney X rays during pregnancy. Today, ultrasonography can often provide the required information without radiation. The stone may be passed spontaneously, or a urologist will have to remove it.

Leg Cramps. It is terribly disconcerting: You awaken from a dream to feel your calf suddenly clenching as though you'd been running a marathon. You can nudge your husband awake for an emergency massage and clench your teeth until the pain goes away. Or you can alleviate the pain by straightening your leg and slowly flexing your foot, so that your heel is pushed forward and your toes point at the ceiling. In fact, doing this exercise before you go to sleep may prevent leg cramps from occurring.

If stretching or massage helps the pain subside, you can use a warm heating pad or compresses to provide further comfort. But if pain persists, notify your practitioner. In some cases, leg cramps indicate the presence of blood clots (thrombophlebitis) and require medical attention. Treatment usually consists of medication and bed rest (or, much less usually, surgery).

The most common cause of leg cramps is a calcium-phosphorus imbalance, an indication that you may not be drinking enough milk. Downing three to four glasses every day during pregnancy should provide enough calcium. If you have difficulty digesting milk or simply do not like it, you may need to take calcium supplements. But still do partake of alternative sources of calcium, such as other dairy products (yogurt, cheese), canned salmon or sardines with bones, broccoli and other cooked fresh greens (collards, kale, turnip greens).

Liver Changes. Tests of liver function change in pregnancy due to substances coming from the placenta. Because circulatory estrogen is increased, the palms of a pregnant woman's hands get red, and "spiders," little red marks on the body, which are not normally seen unless someone has liver disease, are quite common and normal during pregnancy.

Loss of Support in the Pelvic Area. In some women, increased abdominal pressure exerted by the growing uterus or the force of labor can weaken the ligaments and muscular support of the pelvic structures, causing a pelvic organ to fall down or slip from its proper position. Older age, heredity, cigarette smoking, and diseases such as asthma and diabetes increase a woman's likelihood of developing this problem. Loss of support in the pelvic area includes such problems as:

- *Cystocele*, the descent of the urinary bladder
- *Urethrocele*, slippage of the passage leading from the bladder to the outside of the body
- *Uterine prolapse*, the descent of the uterus through the vaginal tract, even to the point where the cervix or even the entire uterus may come down to or through the vaginal opening
- *Enterocele*, a hernia in which bowel encased in peritoneal lining descends, putting pressure on the top of the vagina
- *Rectocele*, descent of the rectum so that it causes the adjacent vaginal wall to bulge through the vulva

Symptoms include a heavy feeling in the pelvic area, pressure on the bladder or bowel, and protrusion of the vaginal wall. Loss of urine may occur during activities that increase abdominal pressure, such as straining, coughing, lifting, and laughing. This condition is called *urinary stress incontinence*.

In the event of cystocele or urethrocele, Kegel exercises (see page 182) may help urinary stress incontinence by strengthening a secondary set of muscles that control urine spillage. However, Kegels cannot restore the essential angle between bladder and urethra that keeps urine from spilling.

If a problem with descent of the pelvic organs persists, corrective surgery can be performed. This is best done after a woman has had all the children she wants, since another pregnancy following surgery could cause the problem to recur.

Lungs and Shortness of Breath. One day in her third trimester, a woman was walking up a familiar hill with her husband when he noticed her huffing and puffing. "You're getting out of shape," he said. "No, it's the effect of the shape I'm in!" she replied. As your uterus extends upward, it crowds your lungs. You might feel yourself not exactly gasping for air, but feeling the need to slow down so you can breathe more easily. Keeping your posture straight can aid your breathing by giving your lungs more room to expand.

Shortness of breath is unlikely to mean you are short of oxygen, since oxygen consumption increases in pregnancy, reflecting the increased requirement. And relief will come: A few weeks before you give birth, the fetus will probably "drop" lower into your pelvis, a shift that positions it for birth. The drop, also called "lightening," eases pressure on your lungs.

Miscarriage. Many women worry about miscarriage, especially during the first trimester, when it is most common. In many cases, miscarriage occurs very early at approximately the time when a menstrual period should come, or slightly after that. In this situation, called *subclinical abortion*, a woman often does not even know she is pregnant; she experiences heavier-than-usual bleeding that she might interpret as a heavy period that is several days late, but is actually the "products of conception" being passed.

What is commonly recognized as miscarriage occurs after pregnancy is diagnosed. At least half of all miscarriages occur because the embryo is defective. Miscarriage might be called nature's way of preventing the birth of babies who would not be able to survive, or whose health would be severely compromised.

Yet though miscarriage may be a merciful event, it is an emotionally traumatic one as well. It is the loss of the child that would have been; it is the end of hopes and dreams, at least for now. The experience also raises the specter of future pregnancies coming to the same sad end. One miscarriage does not necessarily predict another, and most women do sustain healthy pregnancies and births following miscarriage.

There are, however, specific factors associated with a higher risk of miscarriage.

- *Abnormal genetic traits, hormonal imbalances, or disease* (including herpes and other sexually transmitted and systemic diseases) can be diagnosed by such means as cultures, antibody studies, and various blood tests for hormonal levels. Infections can often be eradicated by antibiotics, and hormonal disturbances, such as thyroid disorders, can also be treated with the appropriate medication.

- *Abnormalities of the reproductive organs,* such as a septate uterus (a congenital condition in which the uterus is divided into two parts), scarring, adhesions (Asherman's syndrome), or a misshapen uterus due to fibroids, can be diagnosed through examination of the uterus with an instrument called a hysteroscope. The hysteroscope not only diagnoses such problems; it also corrects some. For example, it can sometimes be used to remove a septum or fibroids. Scarring and Asherman's syndrome are major causes of infertility.

Fibroids, benign uterine tumors that rarely cause miscarriage, can also be diagnosed through hysteroscopic examination or ultrasonography. Subcutaneous fibroids that impinge on the lining of the uterus can be shaved down by an instrument introduced through a hysteroscope.

- *Older maternal (and possibly paternal) age* increases miscarriage risk.
- A *cervix that cannot stay closed* can threaten the pregnancy's ability to proceed. The condition, labeled an *incompetent cervix*, can occur in the second or third trimester. Treatments include bed rest, surgically suturing the cervix closed until the pregnancy reaches term, and medication to prevent uterine contractions.
- *Cigarette smoking* not only increases the risk of miscarriage; it also can lead to low birth weight and respiratory and other problems.

MISCARRIAGE WARNING SIGNS. Immediately notify your practitioner if you experience one or both of the following:

- *Vaginal bleeding*, whether in the form of spotting, pink or brown discharge, or copious bleeding.
- *Cramping*, whether or not accompanied by bleeding.

Mood Swings. If you feel down for no apparent reason, or if you feel an equally inexplicable rush of joy, pregnancy hormones may be the cause. Knowing that mood changes are common during pregnancy should help you cope with them, even stand back a bit and "watch" the moods instead of feeling swept up by them.

Multiple Fetuses. Twins, triplets, quadruplets? You are more likely to have multiples if you or your partner are a twin or have a family history of twins, but the advent of fertility drugs has made multiple fetuses more common. Drugs stimulate the ovaries to produce more eggs, so more have a chance of being fertilized and implanted. *In vitro* fertilization (laboratory insemination of eggs usually with the husband's sperm and sometimes with donor sperm) also increases the chance of multiple fetuses, since more than one fertilized egg is usually implanted in the uterus to increase the odds of success.

Multiples are usually diagnosed when your practitioner feels the uterus is bigger than it should be for the length of gestation, hears more than one heart beating, or feels more than one head or buttocks. Unusually large weight gain may alert your practitioner to suspect twins. Ultrasound provides confirmation of the diagnosis and a more precise count. Identical twins (33 percent of all twins) are created when one fertilized ovum divides in half. The remainder are fraternal twins, the result of separate eggs being fertilized and implanting at about the same time.

Learning that you are carrying twins (or more) requires an instant revision in your vision of motherhood: double vision. Like others before you, you will find a way to feed, clothe, diaper, rock, and stroll two (or more) babies simultaneously. More to do, more to love. And your children will have built-in playmates, a real boon as they get older. It can be exhausting to care for two or more babies, but many couples cannot imagine anything better. "An instant family," one man called it. "Two kids at the same time: how efficient!"

But before you shop for double strollers, consider how having multiples affects your pregnancy.

- *Diet.* For each additional fetus you are carrying, add 300 calories to your daily pregnancy diet. Expect to gain closer to forty pounds instead of the usual twenty to thirty. Take a prenatal vitamin/mineral supplement.
- *Exercise.* Many practitioners recommend that you keep exercise gentle, and primarily rest during the third trimester. Multiples are frequently premature; avoiding exertion helps avert early labor.

- *Labor and Childbirth.* Many women deliver twins vaginally, if both twins are coming headfirst. However, if one fetus is presenting as a breech, or if there are triplets or more, cesarean section is often needed.

Nails. All that oxygen-rich blood circulating through your body stimulates your nails to grow faster. Calcium in the three to four glasses of milk you drink every day helps nails look especially healthy. Dry, brittle nails during pregnancy may attest to insufficient calcium intake. You might be worried that your bones, too, are suffering from lack of calcium. Your fetus will take the calcium it needs; it's up to you to make sure you meet your own body's needs.

Nausea and Vomiting. Many a pregnant woman could, like Sartre, write a book titled *Nausea*, about the queasy sensation that comes "as an illness does . . . cunningly, little by little," making one feel "a little strange, a little put out." Euphemistically called "morning sickness," nausea is often an early symptom of pregnancy. It is a misnomer, too: Come noon, "morning" sickness sometimes lingers on, even into evening. And though you may hear that morning sickness is "supposed to" be confined to the first trimester, it may last through the second and even into the third, although it usually doesn't.

Nausea may be followed by vomiting as well, most commonly in the first trimester but sometimes well beyond. One woman, afflicted with nausea and vomiting throughout her pregnancy, tried many antidotes—from switching toothpaste brands, to nibbling on rice cakes, to avoiding anything with tomato sauce. She got her hopes up when something worked, then became discouraged when nausea returned. She became so accustomed to nausea and vomiting as part of her daily life that she could not imagine ever being digestively calm again. What a relief it was when, the day after giving birth, she was able to down orange juice with breakfast and enjoy spaghetti marinara for dinner. Birth ended nausea, and she could eat again without fearing its return.

Theories abound about why nausea occurs during pregnancy, and why some women feel it and others do not. It may be associated with an increased level of hCG, the pregnancy hormone, or with digestive-tract changes. In a circular catch-22 of pregnancy, nausea may even be made worse by excess stomach acid if a woman does not eat because of nausea.

One theory proposes that nausea is an emotional response to feelings of ambivalence or distress about a pregnancy. For some women, that may be true, and you might consider whether you have such feelings that you need to express and work through. But don't let the theory make you feel even worse. Nausea is not a litmus test of motherliness. Queasiness at the sight of manicotti does not necessarily reveal underlying emotional turmoil. It may just mean: Skip the manicotti.

There are several things you can do to banish nausea—but do *not* take antinausea drugs. Especially during the first trimester, your fetus's major organ systems are being formed, and it is better not to introduce any drugs into your own system.

Here is what you *can* do:

- *Eat a few saltine crackers or rice cakes*, especially first thing in the morning. You might want to keep some by your night table and eat them even before you get out of bed. Putting something in your stomach right away can short-circuit nausea.
- *Eat smaller, frequent meals* instead of three large ones. The press of your uterus on your stomach can hamper digestion of large quantities of food. Smaller meals are easier to digest, and eating more often does not give stomach acids a chance to accumulate.
- *Become your own detective.* Figure out which foods or sub-

stances (like a particular brand of toothpaste or mouth-wash, for example) bring on nausea, and avoid them. Don't bother being "logical." It does not matter if you have always loved Chinese food or spicy barbecue; if these foods bother you now, shun them until the baby is born.

If you are vomiting often:

- *Tell your practitioner* so he or she can monitor whether you and the fetus are getting enough nourishment. If you cannot keep any food down at all, for days at a time, you may need intravenous feeding.
- *Take prenatal vitamin and mineral supplements* prescribed by a physician to ensure that you and the fetus are getting sufficient nutrients, particularly iron and folic acid. You may also need a special diet.
- *Drink lots of water* to replace fluids you lose through vomiting.

Nosebleeds and Congestion. Nosebleeds sometimes occur in pregnancy, especially if nasal membranes are dry due to winter heat, or tender due to a cold. Using a humidifier may help. If you have a nosebleed, do not tilt your head back, since blood could seep back down your throat and make you gag. Instead, lean slightly forward and squeeze the bleeding nostril or nostrils. Apply firm but gentle pressure for three to five minutes, and breathe through your mouth. If bleeding persists or if nosebleeds occur frequently, call your practitioner.

Pregnancy hormones that cause soft tissues to swell also affect the nose. Congestion and postnasal drip are also common during pregnancy. Keep air moist with a humidifier, drink plenty of water and orange juice, and avoid blowing your nose hard. A little petroleum jelly inserted into the nostrils can keep your nose from getting sore and raw.

Placenta Problems. Pregnancy is about the relationship between the woman and the fetus, but the placenta plays a crucial supporting role; without it, there is no pregnancy. The placenta must implant in the right way, in the right position, and must grow and flourish right alongside the fetus, for the duration of the pregnancy. It must not detach from the uterine wall, or be located over the cervical os (the cervical opening), or age prematurely, or become infected. If any of these conditions occurs, birth complications can arise.

- *Placenta previa* is the location of the placenta so low in the uterus that it wholly or partially blocks the cervix, which is the exit to the vagina. The condition may occur more frequently in multiparous women (women who have been pregnant several times).

  Cesarean section is necessary in most cases of partial blockage and all cases of full blockage.
- *Abruptio placenta* occurs when a placenta prematurely loses its secure mooring on the uterine wall and can no longer transmit vital oxygenation between woman and fetus. The condition usually occurs late in pregnancy, causes bleeding, and can be life-threatening for both woman and fetus. Immediate delivery, often through cesarean section, is required.
- *Intrauterine growth retardation* happens when the placenta inadequately transmits the nutrients the fetus needs. The condition may be caused by cigarette smoking during pregnancy or by various disease processes including diabetes.

Postterm Pregnancy. If your due date has come and gone, you may worry that you will be pregnant forever. You imagine tabloid headlines: WOMAN CONTINUES WORLD'S LONGEST HUMAN PREGNANCY, WINNING MATERNITY CLOTHES ASSOCIATION'S "BEST CUSTOMER AWARD." Or might you even qualify for the Longest

Mammal Pregnancy, bypassing Baird's beaked whale (gestation: 519 days) and the African elephant (twenty-two to twenty-four months)?

You must be tired of daily requests by friends and relatives for an up-to-the-minute report: "Well? Any action yet?" If you have other children, you might explain the delay by reading them Fran Manushkin's delightful picture book *Baby, Come Out*, about a family's hilarious efforts to persuade a baby to leave the cozy womb and come out and join them.

Remember that due dates are only approximate. Delivery two weeks before or after is still on time. Beyond two weeks can be a significant problem, unless it simply indicates a miscalculation of when you conceived. Discuss the situation with your obstetrician.

The fundamental issue is the condition of the fetus and placenta. Some postterm fetuses continue to thrive in the uterus— the only disadvantage being that they may become too large to delivery vaginally. However, the placenta is a time-limited organ, designed to expire after its nine-month term of service. Like a *Mission Impossible* tape, the organ begins to self-destruct by the end of pregnancy. An aged placenta cannot support the fetus's continued growth.

Two effective tests employing the fetal monitor can determine whether the fetus is thriving. The nonstress test, done with an external fetal monitor, confirms that the fetal heart responds appropriately by accelerating its pace in response to fetal movements. If the nonstress test is not reassuring, then a contraction stress test may be done. This stress test assesses the fetal heart's response not to its own movements, but to simulated uterine contractions. If the fetal heartbeat does not falter and responds appropriately in either test, the fetus is judged not to be under stress and is presumed capable of withstanding the stress of labor.

Another valuable evaluative procedure is the fetal biophysical profile, performed by combining ultrasonography and the fetal heart monitor. The doctor observes the amount of amniotic fluid and the fetus's movement, muscle tone, and breathing movements.

On the basis of these tests and other evidence, your practitioner will be able to decide whether and when to induce labor.

Premature Rupture of Membranes ("Bag of Waters"). The fluid-filled amniotic sac usually breaks during labor, but sometimes a trickle of liquid is the first sign the labor has begun. Many women fear embarrassment if membranes rupture in public, using the sudden gush and splat of a water balloon as their point of reference. It does not usually happen that way, because the fetus's head blocks the flow of fluid from the cervix. You might want to wear a sanitary pad around your due date just in case. And if a puddle *does* form, try to take it in stride and calmly ask for assistance. Most people are happy to help a pregnant woman in need.

If you are near due date and the fetus's lungs are mature, then ideally you should deliver within twenty-four hours. However, days, even weeks, can safely be allowed to elapse between membrane rupture and birth if the membranes ruptured while the fetus's lungs are still immature. In such cases, care must be taken to keep the uterus infection-free by making sure nothing penetrates the vagina (that means no sexual intercourse, no routine vaginal examinations, etc.) and by taking frequent white blood cell counts and amniotic-fluid cultures.

Preterm Labor need not always result in premature birth. Frequently medications such as ritodrine can be used to stop preterm labor, and in some cases bed rest alone is effective. Early diagnosis of threatened preterm labor is extremely important. This requires regular prenatal-care visits, prompt reporting of any contraction activity to your practitioner, and, if necessary, contraction monitoring at home or in the hospital.

Premature birth must be avoided whenever possible because

fetuses benefit from every moment they stay in the uterus through the ninth month. Neonatologists can keep premature babies alive at ever-earlier ages, but the infants' immature lungs often cause serious respiratory problems.

Rh Incompatibility. The Rhesus (Rh) factor is a blood component that most people have and some lack. Whether you have it or not does not affect your own health. But a problem does exist if you are Rh-negative and your fetus is Rh-positive (reflecting its father's Rh-positive genes). Your body experiences the fetus's Rh factor as a foreign matter that must be fought off and produces antibodies that cross the placenta and demolish the fetus's red blood cells. The fetus becomes anemic and is in danger of still-birth. Jaundice is the result of the destruction of fetal red blood cells.

An Rh-negative woman's first pregnancy is often problem-free. But as she delivers the first baby, some of the baby's blood may get into the woman's circulation, and her body will recognize it as a foreign substance. Then, with each subsequent pregnancy, antibodies produced against the fetal blood attack and destroy the fetal red blood cells.

Ironically and wonderfully, the birth of one Rh-positive baby qualifies a woman to receive a treatment that will protect future pregnancies. An injection of Rhogam (Rhesus gammaglobulin) during pregnancy as suggested by the doctor and within seventy-two hours after the Rh-positive baby's birth destroys fetal blood cells that remain in the mother's blood and keeps her from producing antibodies. Repeating the procedure after each subsequent birth, miscarriage, or abortion maintains her antibody-free status. Because of this, very few Rh-negative women get antibodies that interfere with pregnancy.

Even if they do get antibodies, several medical interventions enable many Rh-negative women to produce healthy babies. Rh titers are blood tests given to a pregnant woman to determine whether and to what extent she is producing Rh antibodies.

Amniocentesis with evaluation of the amniotic fluid determines whether the fetus is significantly affected. Timely induced labor may preserve enough of a fetus's red blood to see it through the birth process. If the fetus is anemic, it can be given a transfusion while it is still inside the uterus. After birth, transfusing the fetus with Rh-negative blood can often save its life.

Rubella (German Measles). Children today are inoculated against rubella, but many adults have never had the disease or the vaccine. If you have not had either, it is best to get inoculated against rubella before embarking on pregnancy; you must wait at least three months after inoculation before you try to conceive.

If you are already pregnant and are not sure whether you are immune to rubella, your practitioner will do a rubella-titer test during your first prenatal visit. A negative result means that you are not immune and must be vigilant about avoiding any exposure to the disease during your pregnancy, since rubella can cause severe birth defects. A famous Agatha Christie murder mystery, in fact, centers around an actress's bitter resentment of a woman from whom she contracted rubella while pregnant; the actress sought revenge for her baby's birth defects.

After you give birth, request the rubella vaccine and wait at least three months before conceiving again.

Saliva Excess. You may notice that your salivary glands seem to be working overtime. Increased saliva is an annoying, occasionally nauseating side effect of pregnancy, but should not be a major problem. If it bothers you a lot, discuss the situation with your practitioner.

Sciatic Pains. These sharp, skewering sensations run down the buttocks into the legs, and are caused by the uterus's pressure on the sciatic nerve. Relieve pains by shifting your position, applying warm (not hot) compresses or heating pad, or by lying on your back with knees raised. Consult a physician to ensure there is no disk disease that can cause permanent nerve damage.

Sexually Transmitted Diseases (STDs). Many women are unaware that they are infected with STDs, such as HIV (the human immunodeficiency virus that causes AIDS), gonorrhea, chlamydia, or syphilis. Some STDs can exist within the body for a long period of time and cause damage without causing symptoms, especially in women, who can unwittingly transmit them to a fetus. If you have any reason to believe that you or your partner may have been exposed to STDs, recently or even years ago, ask your practitioner to order tests for as wide a range of STDs as possible. Do not be embarrassed; many women take this precaution, and your practitioner has heard the request many times before.

If tests reveal that you are infected with an STD, discuss the implications and options with your practitioner. Here are some facts you should know:

- *Chlamydia* can be transmitted from woman to fetus. For this reason, erythromycin ointment or similar treatments are used protectively for the baby's eyes at the time of birth to prevent eye infection.
- *Cytomegalovirus* (CMV) scarcely affects a woman but can cause birth defects. It is not necessarily a sexually transmitted disease, since it may be spread through the respiratory tract as well as through the genital tract, bladder, and breasts. There is no known treatment.
- A *gonorrhea culture* should be standard procedure during every woman's pregnancy. Untreated gonorrhea is not believed to hinder fetal development, but it can be transmitted during the fetus's passage through the birth canal, causing blindness. Today, in every hospital birth (and,

one hopes, in home births), practitioners prevent blindness by using antibiotics such as erythromycin ointment
into the newborn's eyes. The procedure is safe and a good
example of wise preventive medicine.

- *Herpes* can increase your likelihood of miscarriage and
premature delivery. During passage through the birth canal, the baby can contract the virus if you have active
sores, placing the child at risk of brain damage and death.
Delivering by cesarean section keeps the child healthy by
avoiding any contact with sores. However, many women
with herpes can and do safely deliver vaginally if they are
carefully monitored to make sure that no active sores are
present. Throughout the ninth month, have regular Pap
smears and viral cultures to determine whether the virus
is currently dormant or active. A negative culture within
three days of delivery suggests that vaginal delivery would
be safe, but this must be confirmed with your practitioner.
After the baby is born, continue to protect its health by
making sure the baby does not have any direct contact
with active sores in the future. (For example, if you have
active sores, do not take a bath with your baby or let it
sit on your lap if you are unclothed.)

- *HIV*, the virus that causes acquired immune deficiency
syndrome (AIDS), can be transmitted from woman to
fetus. Discuss the possibility of transmission with your
practitioner. Consider whether the risk is acceptable to
you, since a child who develops AIDS may live a relatively
brief life and experience pain and suffering.

- *Human papilloma virus* causes genital warts. The warts will
not affect the baby *unless* you use podophyllin to treat
them; it can be absorbed through the skin and damage
the fetus.

- *Syphilis* should be routinely tested for at your first prenatal
visit. It can cause birth defects or stillbirth. The fetus may

suffer no ill effects, however, if syphilis is detected and treated early in pregnancy, within the first trimester.

Skin Changes. That famed pregnancy "glow" is not automatically yours. Increased blood circulation can bring a lovely rosiness to your complexion, but it won't do you much good if you don't take care of yourself. Your skin tells all. Every fresh salad you eat, every night you go to bed early, every invigorating swim or walk, every glass of water you drink, and every stress-busting meditation session do add up to a healthy radiance.

Following are common skin problems and how to cope with them:

- *Blotches, blemishes, and excessively dry or oily skin* often occur during pregnancy, thanks to those ever-active pregnancy hormones. Good skin care can make a difference. Remove makeup every night with a gentle makeup remover or baby oil. Keep skin clean with a mild soap, plentiful rinsing with warm water, and "steam cleaning." Plug the drain in your sink and run hot water. Lean over the sink and let the steam gently rise to your face. Drape a towel over your head as a tent to help contain the steam. Do not get too close, though—and remember to come up for air so you won't get dizzy!

  If your skin is dry, apply moisturizing cream in the morning and at bedtime after you wash your face. Also moisturize hands, elbows, knees, and ankles, which can also develop dry patches.

  For oily skin, thorough cleansing using a rough washcloth and use of a mild astringent, like witch hazel, help clear pores of grease. Persistent acne may be due to inadequate makeup removal or cleaning or to poor diet, stress, and inadequate rest.
- *"Spiders"* are tiny distended blood vessels that look like

fine, raised red asterisks. Hormonal changes cause them, and they usually vanish after delivery. They generally appear on the face, neck, upper chest, and arms, and can be covered with makeup if you wish.

- *The pregnancy mask* is a pattern of smooth brown or yellowish patches on the forehead and cheekbones. Like "spiders," it vanishes when pregnancy ends. If it bothers you, experiment with using two shades of makeup on your face to conceal it. A visit to a makeup specialist may provide a helpful introduction to new products and techniques.
- *Shiny skin* is part of that beautiful pregnancy glow. But maybe, like Rudolph the Red-Nosed Reindeer, you feel you are glowing too conspicuously. A light dusting of translucent powder can mute the shine. Bright red lipstick can accentuate shine, so try brown- or plum-colored tones.
- *Are you a brunette raccoon?* Dark-haired women sometimes develop sooty marks under their eyes that make them look as though they haven't slept in weeks. Under-eye concealers do the trick.
- *Stretch marks* occur partly because of hormones and partly because stretched skin shows the stress. To a degree, they are genetically determined. You may be able to minimize them by keeping weight gain within twenty to thirty pounds, and by keeping skin supple through a good diet. Massaging cocoa butter or lanolin cream onto your abdomen, breasts, and thighs feels good and softens skin but will not prevent stretch marks. Try not to lament them too much. First of all, they look most prominent after childbirth, and eventually fade to a subtle silvery white. But more important, your body does not have to look like a young teenager's in order to be beautiful and sexy. Stretch marks are a sign of experience, a souvenir (welcome or not) of creating new life. If you don't let them bother you, your partner will hardly notice or mind them.

- *The linea nigra* is a brown-pigmented line that extends from the pubic hair to the navel in some pregnant women. Sometimes it fades after pregnancy and sometimes it doesn't. As with stretch marks, it is a matter of attitude: Many people feel that the *linea nigra* looks very sexy peeking out over a bikini bottom.

Teeth and Gum Changes. Good teeth depend on adequate calcium, especially during pregnancy, when the fetus's needs for the mineral are great. If you drink three to four glasses of milk per day (or get sufficient calcium from the other sources described in this book's section on diet), your teeth will stay strong and healthy.

Overall swelling of tissues during pregnancy affects gums, which may be sensitive and bleed more easily. Do not overpamper them, however, because it can make the situation worse. Brush teeth at least twice a day, angling the toothbrush to brush the teeth where they meet the gums. Run the brush over your tongue, too, to help keep breath fresh. Floss daily to keep teeth clean and to prevent gum infection.

Visit your dentist at least once during pregnancy. Tell your dentist you are pregnant and that you wish to avoid X rays and anesthesia. However, if you have any cavities or infections, it is best to detect and treat them right away, so infection does not spread and cause any problems for you or your fetus. If an anesthetic is necessary, ask your dentist to use local anesthetic. Wear a lead apron for shielding if you must have X rays.

Toxoplasmosis. It is your partner's turn to clean the cat's litter box—and your turn won't roll around again until your baby is born. Parasites found in cat feces and raw or very rare meat can transmit toxoplasmosis. In adults, the infection causes only mild symptoms—faint rash, slight fever, perhaps swollen glands, all no-big-deal symptoms that often pass unnoticed. When transmitted to a fetus, however, toxoplasmosis can cause birth defects or death. Women who test positive for the infection may want to consider terminating the pregnancy.

You do not necessarily have to find a new home for your own cats, although that would be ideal. Have them tested. If they are infection-free, make sure they stay that way by keeping them indoors, away from other cats or animals. Infected cats should stay at a kennel.

Avoid strays and other people's cats and never handle cat litter. Only eat meat that has been cooked at least medium, and do not give raw meat to your cats, either. If you have a garden, wear gloves as a precaution against any feces cats may have excreted there.

Urination/Bladder Control. Pressure on the bladder from the weight of the fetus is only one reason pregnant women urinate more frequently—and certainly early in pregnancy when the fetus weighs so little, it is not a factor at all. Hormones cause increased urination early in pregnancy. And because you have an increased blood volume, you have more fluid to excrete, both your own waste products and those of the fetus.

Increased urination, though it may be a nuisance, should not be painful, and the urine should be clear, never bloody. If you ever do experience pain or bleeding, notify your practitioner at once. Among the problems the symptoms may indicate, the most common during pregnancy is cystitis (urinary-tract infection), which can be treated with medication that does not affect the fetus.

Some pregnant women, especially those who have had several pregnancies, experience *stress incontinence*, the leakage of urine when they cough, laugh, lift objects, or exercise. It is annoying but correctable. Ask your practitioner for exercises that can tighten the muscles in the bladder area. Among these are Kegel exercises: When you urinate, tighten your bladder muscles in order to stop the flow of urine for a moment, then release to let the urine out. Do the exercise every time you urinate, to develop the habit of strengthening those muscles. The exercise is also good for toning vaginal muscles.

Exercises help most women, and certainly after delivery incontinence should go away completely. If it persists, you may decide to have surgery to elevate the neck of the bladder back into its proper position.

Uterine Atony is the uterus's failure to contract after the baby is delivered, causing postpartum hemorrhage, sometimes at the site on which the placenta grew. Hemorrhage is treated with drugs that cause uterine contractility and blood transfusions, if necessary.

Vaginal Discharge and Infection. Vaginal discharge increases during pregnancy. The pale, mucuslike discharge may have a distinctive but not unpleasant odor, and should not cause any problems. If you do experience burning, itching, redness, swelling, or if the discharge becomes foul-smelling, frothy and yellowish, or white and cheesy, chances are you have one of the vaginal infections so common during pregnancy: candida or yeast infection (moniliasis). Do not try to treat it on your own. Your practitioner needs to diagnose precisely which type of infection you have and prescribe the appropriate vaginal cream or suppository. The medication will not harm your fetus and will provide prompt relief for you.

Varicose Veins. Leg veins have valves that can malfunction under pressure and allow blood to flow backward, causing soft blue bulges known as varicose veins. Pregnancy is a source of great pressure on the legs. Varicose veins can lead to blood clots and inflammation. A blood clot that dislodges and travels through your system is dangerous. It is called an *embolus* and can lodge in a lung. Consult your practitioner if a varicose vein gets red, sore, or hard. However, clots in the superficial veins are rarely dangerous; it is clots in the deep veins of the legs that are much more likely to embolize.

To relieve varicose veins, wear full-leg (not knee-high) support hose, and follow the motto "When up, walk; when down, lie." Standing still or sitting for long periods of time exacerbates varicose veins by allowing blood to stagnate in the lower legs. If your job involves standing for long periods of time, find ways to keep moving, even if you must devise a pretext to move about the room. Teachers: Pace while you lecture. Cashiers: Vary your stance. Clerks: Ask for relief from your post at the counter and walk back to check the stockroom.

When you have a chance to sit down, put your feet up on a footstool, table, or the chair next to you. Elevate feet as often as possible to keep blood flowing back toward the heart.

CHAPTER 10

Looking Into the Future

Q. *What prenatal tests for chromosomal and other abnormalities are available—and how can I decide which, if any, to have?*

Like windows on the future, prenatal tests give you knowledge about the fetus that parents in bygone days could hardly have dreamed of. Tests can alert you to chromosomal abnormalities such as Down syndrome, metabolic disorders, abnormalities such as hemophilia, neural-tube defects such as spina bifida, and other serious problems. Some tests, such as alpha-fetoprotein studies (a blood test) and chorionic-villi sampling, are performed early in pregnancy, but women must wait until the second trimester for amniocentesis, a widely used test.

Who Should Consider Testing?

Prenatal testing can benefit everyone, but especially:

- *Women over thirty-five.* Older women have a higher risk of bearing children with chromosomal abnormalities. Approximately one in every 160 babies born in North America has a chromosomal abnormality. Down syndrome is the most common. The risk of Down syndrome increases steadily as a woman ages: a twenty-year-old woman's chances of having a Down syndrome child is 1 in 1,923; a thirty-five-year-old's is 1 in 365; a forty-five-year-old's is 1 in 32; and a forty-nine-year-old's is 1 in 12. Fifty to 60 percent of spontaneous abortions also show chromosomal abnormalities, lending credence to the long-held belief that a miscarriage can be a blessing in disguise.

- *Couples who have a family history of genetic disorders, or a child with a disorder, or a desire to determine whether one or both is carrying genetic disorders.* Some disorders can be transmitted to the fetus by only one parent. Others are transmitted only when both parents are carriers. Some diseases are particular to certain ethnic populations. These include Tay-Sachs disease, a fatal brain disease, and Gaucher's disease, a blood, spleen, liver, and bone disorder, both of which are carried primarily by Jewish people of Eastern European (Ashkenazi) descent; sickle-cell anemia, a blood disorder carried primarily by black people; and thalassemia, a blood disorder carried primarily by people of Mediterranean descent. Other recessive inherited diseases include cystic fibrosis, a disorder of mucous and sweat glands; galactosemia, a diet-correctable incapacity to digest milk sugar; and phenylketonuria (PKU), a liver-enzyme inadequacy that can cause mental retardation if not caught early. Hospital nurseries routinely test newborns for PKU by drawing a minute amount of blood from their heel. Through this early diagnosis, the test has enabled thousands of children to avoid mental retardation by alerting their parents to dietary modifications that stem PKU's progression.
- *Cousins or other close relatives,* who carry a higher risk of hereditary disorders because of their shared genes.

The Waiting Period

For most couples, prenatal testing is a reassuring experience. But some decry the way having to wait for results makes pregnancy feel conditional. Some women and their partners find themselves emotionally distancing from the pregnancy, not even announcing it to friends and family, buying maternity clothes, or daring to fantasize about the baby prior to testing. They feel: Why get our hopes up, or anyone else's, until we know this is a "go-ahead" pregnancy that will get carried to term? Good test results are a relief and a release. Sprung from first-trimester limbo, the couple now feel free to savor pregnancy's remaining months.

But many people do not have such qualms. They do announce the pregnancy right away; they do proceed with confidence that a healthy baby will be born. Perhaps it is a measure of faith or optimism.

When the Test Reveals Fetal Problems

When test results indicate problems, retesting may be necessary to rule out a "false positive." If retesting confirms the results, you can decide whether to terminate or continue the pregnancy. A genetic counselor can help guide you and your partner through the decision-making process by discussing the range of problems the child could face, the possible emotional and financial costs for you and other family members, and support resources to which you could turn if you decide to continue the pregnancy.

For some people, there is no decision to make: They will not choose abortion under any circumstances. Although it is unquestionably easier to raise a healthy child, many children with medical problems have become beloved and treasured members of the family. Couples who decide to continue the pregnancy can use the time before birth to research the disorder, connect with support groups, and prepare themselves and other family members for the challenges—and joys—ahead.

Preventing and Treating Fetal Problems

There are various means to prevent fetal disorders during pregnancy. For example, where there is Rh incompatibility between woman and fetus, a blood transfusion can be performed even while the fetus is still *in utero* by transfusing blood through the umbilical cord. Diabetic women can prevent fetal complications by diligently watching their diets and monitoring their blood-glucose levels and insulin needs. Avoiding alcohol and cigarette smoking are two of the most important ways to prevent fetal damage.

For some fetal problems, there is the option of fetal therapy, the correction of certain fetal disorders prior to birth. For example, intrauterine surgery has been used to install tiny tubes into the malfunctioning bladders of fetuses to enable them to drain normally, thus averting kidney damage. Ultrasonography provides a crucial guide.

While fetal therapy can offer hope for once-hopeless cases, treatments are often experimental and involve certain risks to the mother and/or the fetus. Treatment may:

- endanger the woman's own health
- be successful, but the fetus may have other problems that are irreparable or detectable only after birth
- be unsuccessful, or only partially successful, or prove traumatic and cause the fetus to die
- induce premature labor
- cause side effects, now or in the future, that, because the treatment is experimental, are not currently known

Learning the Fetus's Sex

Prenatal tests can also tell you the child's sex. This is most important to know when screening for sex-linked inherited disorders. But most couples are simply curious—and use the information for narrowing down the list of baby names. Others ask not to know, preferring a birthday surprise.

Rarely, people choose to terminate a pregnancy if the gender is not the one they would choose. This situation is one of many that make prenatal testing a thorny ethical issue, as some question whether a woman should have the right to terminate a pregnancy if the child is healthy but of the "wrong" sex.

PRENATAL TESTS

Test/Purpose	What Is Involved	Risk to Woman and Fetus	When Results Are Available
Amniocentesis: Tests for chromosomal abnormalities that could indicate Down syndrome and other disorders. Women over thirty-five have higher incidence. Also reveals fetus's gender	About the sixteenth week of pregnancy, sample of amniotic fluid drawn. Local anesthesia is used, and procedure is guided by ultrasonography.	Small risk of leaking membranes, miscarriage, or, rarely, injury to the fetus from needle.	Results available in two weeks.

Test/Purpose	What Is Involved	Risk to Woman and Fetus	When Results Are Available
Amniocentesis (continued): and (if performed in third trimester) lung maturity. The amniotic fluid is also tested for alpha-fetoprotein to rule out neural-tube defects.			
Chorionic Villi Biopsy (CVB): For chromosomal analysis to detect chromosomal defects.	About the eighth week of pregnancy, small sample of placental cells is obtained through the cervix, guided by ultrasonography.	Slightly higher risk of miscarriage than amniocentesis. Possible increased risk of fetal limb and other defects. Infrequently, possible risk of infection; possible risk of perforation of the uterus.	Results available within one week.

Test/Purpose	What Is Involved	Risk to Woman and Fetus	When Results Are Available
Alpha-fetoprotein (continued): Reveals brain and spinal cord abnormalities (neural-tube defects) such as spina bifida.	Test of woman's blood or amniotic fluid; performed between the sixteenth and eighteenth week of pregnancy.	No risk to woman or fetus from blood test. See information on amniocentesis risks, above.	Results available day after test. Confirmation of abnormalities through amniocentesis and/or ultrasonography recommended due to rate of false positives. Certain malformations may be surgically correctable.
Ultrasonography: Explores reasons for vaginal bleeding, pelvic pain, and frequent miscarriage; confirms gestational age and ectopic pregnancy;	Test performed after fifth week following last menstrual period; woman's bladder must be full to shift uterus into easily viewed position and to	No known risks to woman or fetus.	Results are analyzed immediately.

Test/Purpose	What Is Involved	Risk to Woman and Fetus	When Results Are Available
Ultrasonography (continued): diagnoses missed or incomplete miscarriage, multiple fetuses, hydatidiform mole, fibroids, or other tumors; guides other uterine interventions such as amniocentesis, CVB, and PUBS.	give sonic waves a contrast. Sonography can be done transvaginally, if necessary, in which case the bladder does not need to be full. An amalgam of echoes, represented on a screen as blips, produces a "picture" of the fetus.		
Fetal Blood Sampling (Fetal Serum Assays): Percutaneous umbilical sampling (PUBS) diagnoses sickle-cell anemia, hemophilia, anemia due to	Under anesthesia and via amniocentesis, a needle is inserted into the blood vessels of the umbilical cord	Spasm of umbilical cord could lead to fetal demise.	How soon results are available varies depending on the reason for the procedure.

Test/Purpose	What Is Involved	Risk to Woman and Fetus	When Results Are Available
Fetal Blood Sampling (Fetal Serum Assays) (continued): Rh isoimmunization, and other disorders.	to obtain fetal blood.		
Fetal Skin Sampling: Diagnoses life-threatening dermatologic abnormalities such as epidermolysis bullosa and ichthyosis.	Scrapes small sampling of skin from fetus through a fetoscope.	Risk of miscarriage.	Results available after biopsies are read by a dermatopathologist.

CHAPTER 11

Drugs, Alcohol, Cigarettes, and Caffeine

Q. *Is it safe to take any drugs during pregnancy?*

Never risk your own health and life. Some fetal drug exposure may occur with prescription medications women take to treat life-threatening disorders, such as high blood pressure, diabetes, and epilepsy. This sort of drug exposure is unavoidable, though your doctor will prescribe those medications that will be safest for both you and your fetus.

But over-the-counter and illicit drugs account for a majority of the most commonly reported fetal drug exposures. Many of these drugs are known to be unsafe during pregnancy. Others have not been shown to be safe and should be avoided; they should not be given the benefit of the doubt when a baby's health is at stake. There may be nothing more heartbreaking than the sight of a struggling newborn whose problems were preventable; if its mother had not drunk alcohol, had not taken cocaine, had not taken diet pills, the tiny infant in the incubator would instead be a healthy, thriving baby with a wide-open future. When pregnant women take drugs without a physician's okay, they play Russian roulette with their babies' lives.

Prescription and Over-the-Counter Drugs: Do You Really Need Them?

It is best to avoid all drugs during pregnancy, unless they are drugs prescribed by a physician for life-or health-threatening disorders. And even for ailments that are *not* life-threatening, there *are* certain medications your practitioner can recommend that are not harmful during pregnancy.

But to be on the safe side, become a question-asker. Check with your doctor about any drugs he or she prescribes by asking:

- What risks does this drug pose to the fetus?
- What do I risk if I do *not* take the drug?
- How long has the drug been on the market?
- What has been your experience with other women who have taken it?
- What possible side effects might I experience?
- What specific instructions do I need about how to take the drug? (What time of day, how often, what dosage, for how many days, and should I avoid taking it in conjunction with any specific foods, drinks, other substances?)

Ask the same questions of your pharmacist when considering any over-the-counter (OTC) drug that your practitioner said was all right. (Do not take any OTC drugs without a physician's prior approval.) Read packages carefully. Some over-the-counter medications specifically caution against their use by pregnant women.

Among the types of medications that may cause fetal problems are certain hormones, anticoagulants, antithyroid drugs, chemotherapeutic drugs, metallic substances, antibiotics, antinausea, anticonvulsant, and anti-acne drugs.

The more drug- and alcohol-free your pregnancy is, the more likely you are to give birth to a healthy child. If you are accustomed to medicating yourself when you do not feel well, pregnancy may cause you to reevaluate your response to discomfort. Stoicism is hardly one of our go-get-'em society's favorite traits; it implies a certain degree of passivity, the postponed taking of action to deal with something intolerable. It is the badge of a martyr. Yet when you choose to endure discomfort and forgo drugs during pregnancy, you are being an altruist, not a martyr. You are doing what is best for your fetus's future and therefore your own.

So when you have an ache or a pain that does not absolutely require treatment, try to endure it, or sleep through it, or relax it away with a bath or massage, or even just observe it, instead of turning to medications that could possibly be deleterious to your fetus's health.

Always weigh the benefit of taking the drugs against the possible dangers. For example, acne is not life-threatening for a woman; it is unpleasant, but she can live with it. But some pregnant women have taken Accutane, a prescription vitamin-A compound for the treatment of severe acne, which is associated with malformation of the fetal central nervous system, face, and heart.

A Drug-Free Approach to What Ails You

The packed shelves of the nation's drugstores attest to many people's drug orientation. But if you feel irritable or anxious, for example, do not reach for a tranquilizer or a marijuana joint, but consider:

- Are you getting enough rest?
- Are you eating well?
- Are you stressed-out; do you need to ask for more support from those close to you?
- Is your schedule unrealistically hectic?

- Are you feeling upset, and is this headache the expression of your feelings?
- Would exercising more, or less, be helpful?

Check out all problems with your practitioner to make sure they do not indicate any serious condition. If they do not, then live through your pregnancy as if it is a drug-free zone. No one ever regretted, upon viewing her healthy baby, that she did *not* take that over-the-counter medication or drink that tempting martini on that difficult day in her sixth month.

Q. *I've smoked since I was fifteen. How—and why—should I stop smoking now?*

Many people find it difficult to stop smoking. Nicotine is highly addictive, and the smoking way of life can be, too. Having a cigarette with breakfast in the morning, or while reading the paper, or while talking on the phone, or after having sex, may feel like the inevitable punctuation of the moment, as natural and unquestionable as putting a period at the end of a sentence.

Whether you regard smoking as a pleasure you are loath to give up or as a demon with which you have wrestled unsuccessfully in the past, there is no question that for your fetus, your smoking is a most hazardous habit. When you smoke, you increase your chances of having a premature birth and a low-birthweight baby. Birth weight is important because babies who have intrauterine growth retardation and are delivered underweight for their age of gestation are not as well equipped to cope. They begin life with a deficit, because they have to catch up on weight and strength they should have gained in the uterus.

Smoking constricts blood vessels that carry oxygen to the uterus. This deprives the fetus of oxygen and slows its growth. Smoking also exposes the fetus to carbon monoxide, a toxic gas. Placental abnormalities can also develop. Abruption of the placenta (detachment of the placenta from the uterine wall) is more common in smokers and disrupts the fetus's oxygen supply.

It is an obstetric emergency and is potentially fatal for both woman and fetus.

The effects of smoking even transcend the fetus's birth. The fetus who "smoked" *in utero* becomes a child who is more likely to have respiratory, learning, and behavior problems.

How to Quit. If you have smoked for a long time, quitting may seem like an overwhelming task. When you are trying to adjust to pregnancy, can you handle this life change, too? Yet pregnancy is a wonderful, life-affirming time to quit smoking. You can feel doubly proud of yourself for accomplishing it, because you will improve two lives at the same time. Here are some tips on how to do it:

- Discard any cigarettes you have, and tell your partner and friends that you are quitting and that they should not offer you any more. You might want to start a "Congratulations" fund, in which you put money you would ordinarily spend on cigarettes. After your baby is born, spend the money on something special.
- Use visualization techniques. When you feel like having a cigarette, visualize the fetus holding the cigarette and being surrounded by smoke. Then imagine the cigarette and smoke vanishing, the fetus now healthy. Envision giving birth to a big, healthy baby.
- If you are not ready for "cold turkey," use this more gradual method prior to becoming pregnant: Become aware of the number of hours you can go between cigarettes. Gradually increase the intervals between cigarettes. When you reach six hours, give up smoking completely. Then take it one day at a time. Don't let this process go on too long, though. Have a time frame in mind, a date by which you want to be finished with smoking.
- Sign up for a motivational seminar or consider hypnosis.
- If you miss having a cigarette in your mouth, substitute carrot or celery sticks, a straw, or skinny little pretzels.

- If you don't know what to do with your hands now that you are no longer holding a cigarette, begin a project: needlepoint, knitting, crocheting, mosaic, sketching. Knead dough. Knot macramé. Manicure your nails. Or massage your partner!
- A cigarette can be a way of carving time out of the day; find a new way to do it. For example, if you used to step onto your back porch for a smoke, perhaps it was a way of giving yourself permission to enjoy a few quiet minutes. The burning cigarette would mark time like an hourglass, gradually eroding into ashes until it was time to go inside again. You don't need a cigarette in order to give yourself "breaks."
- Did you feel that a cigarette gave you a "pick-me-up?" Maybe the action of inhaling and exhaling smoke "centered" you. Learn to do it without the cigarette. Some people who meditate simply call it "sitting." Meditation is a time of stillness and quiet, breathing in and out slowly and rhythmically.
- Distract yourself from smoking. Go out with friends who do not smoke, take walks, go to the movies, read.
- Avoid settings that almost beg you to smoke, like bars.
- If your partner smokes, ask him not to smoke around you. This will help you resist joining him, and will protect you and your fetus from "secondhand smoke."

Q. What are the risks if I take illicit drugs while pregnant?

Risks associated with cocaine, heroin, and other drugs are so serious that a woman who uses them is best off postponing pregnancy until she is drug-free and certain she can stay that way. In an ideal world, every pregnant woman would feel no urge for drugs, and every fetus would have a chance from the start of a drug-free life. But if you have become pregnant at a time when you are using drugs, pull together every bit of resolve you can to quit. Find a treatment program. Spend time with people who do not use drugs. Explain to drug-using friends that it is far easier for you to resist using drugs if you are not around them.

Perhaps you envision drug use as a spectrum, with infrequent, "no big deal" smoking of a marijuana joint at one end and heavy cocaine addiction at the other. And perhaps your own drug use is light, and on the more easygoing side of the spectrum, and you do not consider yourself to be in the same league as the addict. But you share the same common denominator: a vulnerable fetus who will be affected, adversely, by any such drugs you take. The fact is, no one knows how much cocaine *or* marijuana may be "safe." Evidence points the opposite way. Marijuana users may have an increased risk of fetal malformations. Cocaine babies have a spate of problems, ranging from potentially fatal detachment of the placenta, to low birth weight, to having to endure the trauma of drug withdrawal in the days after birth. Damage can be lifelong.

Q.   I've heard that alcohol can cause problems during pregnancy. But I always serve wine with dinner. Must I really stop?

A "harmless" glass or two of red wine? It *would* be a delicious accompaniment to sliced steak with mushrooms. The problem is this: It is well established that drinking alcohol when pregnant can cause severe and permanent damage to the fetus. But no one has established just how *little* alcohol is harmful.

Individual differences in how a woman's body processes alcohol may be a factor, though no one knows how to tell in advance of pregnancy which woman is at greater risk. If you drink heavily, try to stop drinking before you conceive or as soon as possible after you become pregnant. Enroll in a treatment program or attend Alcoholics Anonymous meetings. And even if you drink relatively small amounts, stop. The short-term pleasure of a drink is not worth the long-term risk to your child.

Fetal Alcohol Syndrome (FAS) is the most severe form of alcohol-related damage. A child with FAS has one or more of the following problems: low birth weight and size, mental retardation, learning disabilities, abnormally small brain and skull, distinctive facial characteristics (widely spaced, abnormally small eyes; flat cheeks; small, turned-up nose), and heart malformations.

Children whose mothers drank more moderately than FAS babies' mothers can still suffer from Fetal Alcohol Effect (FAE), a group of signs of alcohol-related damage similar to FAS, including low birth weight and size, restlessness, lower than average IQ, and other problems.

If you feel tempted to drink, visualize your fetus holding a wineglass or can of beer. It is a bizarre and disturbing picture—but an accurate one: When you drink, alcohol crosses the placenta. So your fetus is drinking right along with you. You will never regret the drinks you did not take.

Q. *Must I abandon my beloved morning cups of coffee?*

Like brushing teeth and picking up the mail, drinking coffee can be one of life's daily actions. But it is daily with a difference: It is daily because it is addictive.

Heartwarming coffee ads feature friends communing over steaming mugs of java. But the ads don't let on that the smiling, sipping pals would be frowning and jittery if deprived of their caffeine. Nor that a pregnant coffee drinker may risk causing birth defects. Some studies indicate that heavy coffee drinking may cause birth defects, though others disagree. However, it is just common sense that if caffeine, a powerful nerve stimulant, has such a strong effect on adults, it is better not to subject your fetus to it.

Take a week to taper off from caffeine (since sudden complete withdrawal may cause irritability or headaches). Then refrain from it altogether throughout pregnancy and breast-feeding. By then you may be so accustomed to doing without caffeine that you will not even wish to resume. When you do want a hot drink, try heating apple juice or cranberry juice. Avoid teas and colas that contain caffeine.

CHAPTER 12

Home Stretch: The Long, Suspenseful Third Trimester

Q. Should I take childbirth classes?
You *and* your partner will benefit tremendously from the classes, on a number of levels. "Nothing can prepare you for exactly how labor feels," said one woman, "but childbirth classes at least familiarized me with everything else."

Childbirth classes have become a modern-day rite of passage. Their orientation toward preparing not just the woman but the *couple* acknowledges that birth, like conception, involves two people. No matter how supportive a caregiver and nurse, a woman in labor needs the attention and support of someone to whom she is close. If your partner is unavailable for childbirth classes or will not be with you for the delivery, attend classes with another close friend or relative who will serve as your labor partner. Some women have arranged for their mother, best friend, sister, or an independent "labor coach" to be present.

Childbirth classes tell you what to expect during labor and delivery and teach valuable breathing exercises and relaxation techniques. Childbirth educators often make use of helpful teaching aids such as films, charts and drawings, and models that show the birth process.

Classes also give "pregnant couples" an opportunity to meet others and gain support from knowing they are not alone. Such close camaraderie occurs so often that many childbirth classes hold reunions a month or two after the last class. Couples proudly show off their babies, share childbirth tales, and discuss the new thrills, skills, and demands of postpartum life.

Even if you are not sure you want "natural childbirth," enrolling in childbirth classes educates you about all your options— even exploring what anesthesia may be available and whether, how, and when to choose it. Childbirth classes also cover complications that might arise, including cesarean section. Hospital-affiliated classes often provide tours for couples to familiarize them with labor, delivery, and birthing rooms and the maternity ward and nursery. Some also give "sibling" classes to prepare children for the arrival of a new sibling and to show them where they can visit their mother and brother or sister.

The first class can feel momentous—"This is really happening!" Beginning classes elevates the excitement of the third trimester, almost like beginning a countdown toward birth. The timing is perfect: Just when you have more questions, and perhaps more fears, than ever, you join a class whose teacher and other members provide just the information and support you need. Learning breathing techniques may be confusing at first—but by the last class, you will take pride in your mastery of a new respiratory repertoire. And when you walk into the labor room, you will be bolstered by the confidence that comes from being prepared.

Q. How do I select a childbirth class?

Many doctors and nurse-midwives offer classes associated with their practice. These classes of course reflect your practitioner's philosophy and approach, and also usually include a hospital tour.

But if there is a particular approach to childbirth that appeals to you, by all means check out classes that teach it. Just be sure that you discuss your wishes with your practitioner, so that together you can work out any differences in advance.

While "Lamaze" is synonymous with childbirth classes in many people's minds, there are actually several types of classes. All of them seek to educate couples about the labor and birth process, but each has its own angle on how a woman involves herself in the experience.

- *Lamaze technique* focuses on breathing techniques that distract from the intensity of labor contractions. By concentrating on various breathing patterns, a woman can lift her awareness away from the uterus and exert greater control over her childbirth experience. Her labor coach (usually, but not always, her husband) helps remind her which breath to use at various stages of labor and strokes her abdomen with slow, circular motions to help her relax. Lamaze is in some ways a descendant of pioneering work by Grantly Dick-Read in the 1930s. He advocated that women experience greater involvement in childbirth than had previously been the norm.
- *Bradley technique* is more internal; the goal is to avoid distraction. One woman described Bradley as "riding with the contractions." The Lamaze counterpart would be "breathing above the contractions."
- *Kitzinger approach* emphasizes childbirth as part of a woman's sexual continuum. It encourages women to consciously connect with (rather than distance from) labor, in order to focus on the process as a natural and celebratory step in their sexual lives.
- *Leboyer technique* is not a childbirth method but a more humane approach to how the baby is treated once it is born. Frederick Leboyer recommended soft light and warm baths to ease the baby's transition into *ex utero* life. How-

ever, there are instances when brighter light is necessary in order for your practitioner to most safely assist.

Some have even advocated underwater birth, based on the theory that after living nine months in amniotic fluid, the baby would be most comfortable being born into fluid. On the other hand, female whales, who are of course mammals who live and breathe in the sea, do not choose the Leboyer method; they nudge their young to the surface for air. Eventually, your baby will have to breathe like the rest of us, and the underwater approach is neither theoretically nor practically valid.

Shaping Your Own Experience

The above list of childbirth techniques only scratches the surface; there are many more theories of the "right" or "best" way of giving birth. Sometimes new ideas have merit, but sometimes they seem to be well described by the "You Gotta Have a Gimmick" lyrics in the Broadway musical Gypsy.

Any childbirth class should be an enabling experience. That means that it should enable you to feel good about doing your best to get the baby born in the way that is healthiest and safest for both of you. Although drug-free, conscious labor is theoretically the preferred course of action, you should not feel that you "failed" if you needed some pain relief or had a cesarean section. If your experience differs from the "pure" natural childbirth scenario, do not let that diminish your pleasure in seeing your wonderful new baby.

You are just as much a "real woman" and a "good mother" with one means of childbirth as another, when you make your decisions on the basis of what is best for you and your baby. Not for some theoretical woman and her baby—but for you.

Childbirth practitioners—doctors and nurse-midwives alike—are motivated to help you have the best birth experience you can. But always, the most important factor is: *How mother and child can come through the process with the greatest degree of safety and health.*

Checklist: What Childbirth Classes Should Cover

Anatomy—pelvic architecture, the uterus, birth canal, and perineum, placenta, umbilical cord. A three-dimensional model is an especially effective teaching aid.

Stages of Labor—ways in which labor begins, how to know you are in labor and what to do when it starts, how to sustain stamina and focus as labor progresses through the pushing stage.

Breathing Exercises—various techniques for enabling you to actively accept and breathe through contractions (and advice on how to recognize and stop "overbreathing," hyperventilation that can be deleterious).

Labor Coaching—how your labor partner can support you through encouragement, reminders about breathing, serving as your advocate, and helping to make you comfortable.

Labor Monitoring Techniques—how your practitioner follows your progress throughout labor.

Birthing Positions—a review of the various positions in which women give birth, to enable you to choose the one that is most comfortable for you.

Anesthesia—indications, pros and cons, types of anesthesia available and characteristics of each.

Pitocin and Other Labor Aids—indications, pros and cons.

How to Cope with Stress and Anxiety—acknowledgment of the intense emotional roller coaster that pregnancy and labor can sometimes be, with suggestions for how you and your partner can cope.

Cesarean Section—indications, how to prepare for it, how to decide, how to recuperate, how to deal with the emotional impact.

Complications—for both mother and baby, what might occur and how to cope.

Breast-feeding—pros and cons, how to prepare.

Episiotomy—indications, pros and cons, how to prevent, how to recuperate.

Postbirth Events—how baby is evaluated (Apgar score), what baby will look like, bonding and breast-feeding, length of hospital stay, need for support at home.

Sibling Issues—how to prepare children for the arrival of a new sibling.

Q. I want to wait until the baby is born before buying a crib, but my partner is ready to fix up a whole nursery. Am I being needlessly superstitious?

There is no right and wrong answer; do what makes you feel comfortable. The odds are in your favor: Chances are your baby will be fine and will come home from the hospital all set to enjoy its brightly painted room! Optimism is not a misguided emotion; it is an affirmation of the probability that all will go well. But if you feel uneasy about "jumping the gun," take advantage of a service that many baby-furniture and supply stores offer. You can select the crib, changing table, etc., but request that they not be delivered until the baby is born.

In the same spirit, you may welcome having a baby shower while you are still pregnant, or you can ask your friends to schedule it for the month after the baby is born. That way (in case you did not find out the gender in advance of birth) they will know your baby's sex, name—and monogram!

Q. Should I choose a pediatrician now or after birth?
This is one decision you would like to have in place before
the baby is born. Ask your practitioner and friends for recommen-
dations. In making your selection, you might want to meet with
pediatricians in advance (some will do so for free, while others
charge), keeping the following selection criteria in mind:

- *Philosophy and Policies.* For example, are the pediatrician's
  views on breast-feeding versus bottle-feeding similar to
  your own?
- *Rapport and Communication.* Is this pediatrician someone
  you will feel comfortable talking with and asking questions
  of, even "silly" questions (which often turn out not to be
  silly at all)? Some doctors make you feel that they really
  want you to understand what is going on with your child;
  they volunteer explanations and patiently listen to your
  questions and concerns. Other doctors sometimes seem so
  rushed they sound like they are being played at Fast-for-
  ward. They offer few explanations and may seem impatient
  with your questions. This one-foot-out-the-door manner
  does not bother everyone, especially when a pediatrician
  is renowned for his or her expertise. But consider whether
  it will irk *you.*

  Does the doctor have regular call-in times (such as
  between seven and eight in the morning)? Or a reputation
  for calling back quickly when you leave a message? Are
  there other partners in the practice who take over when
  your pediatrician is away?
- *Convenience.* Having a pediatrician within easy walking or
  driving distance (with ample parking available) of your home
  can be a godsend when the weather is bad, or when your
  child has a fever and you want to minimize commuting time.
  If you are going to have to take a crosstown bus and two
  subway trains to get to the doctor, rethink your choice—
  unless the doctor is decidedly superior in other ways.

Also find out what office hours the pediatrician keeps. For working parents who want to accompany their children to medical checkups instead of leaving it to the baby-sitter, evening and weekend appointments meet their needs best.

- *Cost.* Does the doctor accept your insurance plan? Do you have to pay up front, or will the the office bill you or your insurance company?
- *Office Environment.* Is the office clean? Are there books and toys for children to play with while they wait? And how long *is* the average wait? Is the staff warm, friendly, responsive, and well organized?

CHAPTER 13

Labor and Its Sweet Reward

Q. How will I know I am really in labor?

Labor may begin with a whoosh or slow leakage of amniotic fluid when membranes rupture, or with regular contractions that gradually increase in intensity and frequency. They initially occur at ten- to twenty-minute intervals and last about forty-five seconds each. Contractions may feel like a wide pull of sensation across your abdomen or back; early on in labor they are more interesting and exciting than they are uncomfortable. Sometimes they coincide with passage of the "bloody show," which is the mucus plug that seals the cervix during pregnancy. If you have had a baby before, your labor may begin the same way it did then or completely differently.

Call your practitioner when any of these signs of labor occur, and follow instructions about how to time contractions and when to go to the hospital. Depending on how far you live from the hospital, usually practitioners recommend laboring at home until contractions occur five to ten minutes apart. If membranes have ruptured, however, your safest course of action is to call your practitioner and be evaluated at the hospital.

Packing Checklist: What to Take to the Hospital

Warm robe and socks or slippers—Hospitals can be chilly! Make sure the robe is washable since it might get stained.

A *picture or drawing* on which to focus when doing breathing exercises during labor. It might be a photo, or an old postcard, or a drawing, or a mandala—an image that makes you feel serene and spiritually nourished.

Cold pack for use during back labor.

Light, nutritious snacks for your partner (follow your practitioner's advice on how much and whether you can eat, too).

Eyeglasses, if you wear them, and a large mirror so you can watch your baby being born. (The hospital probably has mirrors on hand also.)

Tape recorder and musical tapes to create a peaceful atmosphere during labor.

Washcloth with which your partner can wipe your face.

Lip gloss or petroleum jelly to soothe you if your lips get dry.

A watch with a second hand so you can time contractions.

Massage oil or lotion with which your partner can give you back or leg rubs.

Toiletries—comb and brush, toothbrush and toothpaste, moisturizer (for face, hands, elbows, heels), makeup, deodorant, soap. The hospital will provide sanitary napkins for postbirth discharge. (Do *not* use tampons.)

Books or magazines—for later . . . do not expect to want to read during labor.

A notebook and pen—for jotting down thoughts and feelings, questions for your practitioner, reminders of things for you or your partner to do, lists of baby gifts and thank-you notes to write after you return home.

A camera (and extra film and batteries)—preferably without a flash, for recording this amazing new chapter in your family history.

A list of people for your partner to call and a roll of quarters for the pay phone, a telephone credit card, or a portable phone—

Also, your address book in case you feel like making calls from your hospital room later.

Clothes to wear home—for both you and the baby. Remember, it will take time for your body to return to its prepregnancy shape. So plan on wearing maternity clothes home. For the baby, have two outfits on hand. Cozy baby wear might be a one-piece stretchie with feet or separate booties, a blanket, and a hat (sunbonnet in the summer, warm hat in the winter). If the weather is cold, have a warm quilt or bunting to wrap the baby in. The hospital will provide diapers. If you will travel home by car, remember to provide a car seat for the baby.

Q. What should I expect during labor and delivery?

Labor might be described most simply as a process of dilatation and passage.

Labor's First Stage: Dilatation. Your cervix gradually dilates (opens) so the baby will be able to pass through. A fully opened cervix is ten centimeters, about the size of a large fist. Full dilatation can take hours. Except in very unusual circumstances, labor should not exceed twenty-four hours.

Although the sensations that accompany dilatation are called contractions, you might prefer thinking of them in alternative terms, such as "rushes," "spreading," or "blossoming." These terms remind you that the cervix is expanding, stretching open. When you visualize the cervix widening, you might keep in mind the concentric circles that form when you toss a pebble into a pond. Imagine your cervix gently and steadily opening into a progressively larger circle. Stay patient.

Labor is a journey for the child, but also for the mother—a process of discovery that is uniquely yours. One woman compared labor to the way a plane trip feels like a set-aside time, with the "real world" a distance beneath you. Other women feel a sharp increase in intimacy with their partner, or an unexpected resistance to labor, an impatience to meet the baby, or a dreamlike succession of thoughts and images that made one woman say, "So *this* is what it's like to be inside a kaleidoscope."

An "in-joke" among mothers is the common experience of thinking during labor, "I'll never do *this* again"—only to feel after the baby is born, "This is so wonderful; I want this experience all over again."

"Labor" is aptly named. You work hard on so many levels: to breathe through contractions, to stay focused, to think positive thoughts, to resist the urge to push before you are fully dilated, and at last to push the baby out. Yet throughout there is an edge of exhilaration—the excitement of knowing that the end of labor marks a new beginning. You will have your first face-to-face introduction to the baby you already feel you know so well.

Your experience of labor will be affected by a number of things—how long it takes, how labor progresses, how involved your partner is with you, how encouraging your practitioner and nurses are, how comfortable the setting is, and how free you feel to express your feelings and desires.

Sometimes small things make a difference. One woman felt moved and supported by a tender painting of a mother and baby by Mary Cassatt that hung on the birthing-room wall. Another woman had spent hours over the last month creating a couple of "birthing tapes" and derived great pleasure from playing the music. A third woman felt nourished by the upbeat attitude of a nurse she'd never met before; every time she complained that contractions were getting more intense, the nurse beamed and said, "That's wonderful! It means you're getting closer to having the baby." By showing her a happier way to regard the contractions, the nurse helped the woman stay focused on the goal.

The breathing techniques you learned during childbirth classes help you tolerate contractions, which can be astonishingly intense. Do not worry that you will forget which breaths to use. Your partner and the labor-room nurse will remind you. They can also help make you comfortable through back and leg mas-sage, gentle circular stroking of your abdomen, walking with you, and supporting you in standing, squatting, or reclining positions (whatever is most comfortable for you). You might want to suck on ice chips, or have your partner stroke your face with a moist washcloth, brush your hair, read to you, or lie down with you. Some couples feel that kissing and embracing at times during labor both intensifies the intimacy of the experience and helps labor progress. This can be especially true with nipple stimula-tion, which releases a natural hormone that can speed up labor. However, do not proceed with nipple stimulation unless you get your practitioner's approval.

If labor fails to progress—meaning that you get stuck at a certain level of dilatation—the first course of action (provided that neither mother nor baby shows signs of stress) is simply to wait awhile to see if labor reestablishes itself. Labor does not always chug along like a train on a track. Early on, you may be in the latent phase of labor, which your practitioner will determine. If labor truly stops in the active phase, it might be stimulated (augmented) with oxyto-cin (also known as Pitocin), which stimulates uterine contractions. You can inquire about this option anytime, but remember that your practitioner is trained to know when this is necessary and desirable. Some women dislike the abrupt shift into contractions, since the rhythm is externally rather than internally caused, but others feel relief at getting back into action.

Inducing labor (starting labor when it has not started itself) is also done sometimes when you are over two weeks past your due date (provided that the fetus is not in distress), or when disease or a disabling condition makes prompt delivery medically necessary. If membranes have ruptured and labor has not ensued, labor may need to be induced.

Stage 2: Pushing. When the cervix is fully dilated, the baby can exit the uterus and pass through the birth canal, but it needs you to push it out. You hold your breath and bear down, as you do when you move your bowels. Again, visualization can help you sustain your energy for this demanding task. Even if you do not think you feel the baby moving down much, visualize its onward progress, even if it consists of the most subtle increments.

Some women have the mistaken impression that in two or three pushes, they can get that baby born. While that sometimes happens, the pushing may last far longer than you think. "So near, and yet so far," thought one woman. Her baby had crowned, meaning that the top of its head (its sparse, curly hair) could be seen in the mirror the nurse held. But its journey of only inches would take another hour to accomplish. Do not get discouraged, and do not try to rush it. Push, but also rest between pushes. Tell your practitioner when you need a breather. If your practitioner agrees, try different positions, such as squatting, that may make pushing easier. Specially designed birthing beds and birthing chairs, available in many hospitals and birthing centers, are said to facilitate pushing.

In some instances, though less frequently than in the past, your practitioner may need to help urge the baby through the last part of the birth canal by using forceps (large, gently curving tongs) or a vacuum extractor (a cap applied to the baby's head creates a vacuum, which helps slide the baby out). Needing help does not mean you have "failed" to push adequately. It may be necessary because the baby is large, or you are narrow, or simply that the force you are exerting is not sufficient. Or you may be close to exhaustion, or the second stage of labor (from full dilatation of the cervix) has been sufficiently long, or the baby is starting to show signs of stress.

Your practitioner may perform an episiotomy, a linear incision from the vagina toward (but not into) the anus. An episiotomy can make the baby's passage easier and prevent tearing of the vagina and perineum (the area between the vagina and anus). "Naturally occurring" tears tend to be jagged. If they do not heal properly, you may have uncomfortable scar tissue. Or your vaginal tone may end up being lax, because of a tear interfering

with sexual enjoyment. A properly repaired episiotomy reapprox-
imates the tissues (muscles) of the perineum and closes the vaginal orifice close to its previous size.

After the baby is born, your practitioner (or perhaps your
partner) cuts the umbilical cord. Cutting it fairly soon after
delivery reduces the baby's risk of jaundice.

Do not expect the baby to look like a roly-poly model in a
baby-food ad. A newborn can be on the skinny side, covered
with the cream-cheesy vernix, streaked with blood here and
there. Your practitioner will, if necessary, suction mucus from
the baby's mouth. At one minute and five minutes after birth,
the doctor or nurse-midwife will examine the baby and "score"
its appearance, reflexes, and breathing according to the Apgar
criteria, a means of evaluating newborns. Not long afterward,
you and your partner should be able to hold the baby, and you
can see if it is ready to nurse.

Stage 3: Delivering the Placenta. From five or ten to thirty
minutes after the baby is born, you will deliver the placenta.
Because it is smaller than the baby (and more pliable, since it
contains neither bones nor a large head that must squeeze through
a small space), delivery of the placenta is much easier. Although
you are absorbed in the sight of your new baby, you might wish
to see the placenta. It is like a large slab of liver, but with
distinctive whorls and textures.

Q. *Will I need to be "prepped" for labor?*

The term "prepping" (short for childbirth "preparation") refers to a set of prebirth practices that some women find distasteful
and unnecessary. Once obligatory, they have now become optional or eliminated in many hospitals. If you wish to avoid—or
request—any of them, discuss your wishes with your practitioner
well in advance of labor. Prepping includes:

- *Shaving the pubic area*—The rationale is that it helps prevent infection. But it may actually increase the chance of

infection, in addition to being embarrassing, uncomfortable, and itchy when the hair grows back. Sometimes it is necessary to shave a small area for repair of the episiotomy site.

- *Enema*—This means of emptying the bowels is used to create more usable space in the birth canal for the baby by eliminating feces within the intestines, and to rule out any possibility of contamination from feces expelled during labor, and in some cases to induce labor. But unless a woman has impacted stool, feces are unlikely to interfere with the uterus. And if a bowel movement occurs during labor, stool can quickly be wiped away. For some women, the unpleasantness of an enema counterbalances its theoretical benefits.

Q. Will I need an IV?
Inserting an IV needle in the arm of every pregnant woman is a wise precaution in the event the IV is needed for medication, anesthesia, nutrients, or, less commonly, transfusion. More important, the administration of IV fluids during the hard work of labor prevents maternal dehydration, thereby lessening maternal exhaustion and deleterious effects on the fetus.

Q. Will I need fetal monitoring?
Monitors simply show the heartbeat pattern of the fetus (fetal-heart monitor) and the contraction pattern of the uterus. Your practitioner, a skilled observer, utilizes this constant flow of information as one means of checking the adequacy of your labor and the fetal response to it. Monitors have revolutionized childbirth by providing a technological window through which the fetus's ongoing response to the stress of labor can be evaluated.

External monitors placed on a woman's abdomen record the fetal heart's response to uterine contractions. Internal monitors involve the delicate, shallow insertion of a fine electrode into the fetus's scalp, a procedure that permits the most reliable reading of the fetus's condition. This can be coupled with an internal uterine-pressure monitor, a fine hollow tube that measures the pressure exerted on the amniotic fluid. When the internal monitor indicates stress, the reading can be confirmed by drawing a minute amount of blood from the fetus's scalp and analyzing it for acidity. A low pH, meaning high acidity, indicates asphyxia, which is an inadequate supply of oxygen. The condition reveals that the fetus may not be able to withstand further delay or the stress of vaginal birth. Delivery by cesarean section often is the appropriate form of rescue.

One possible sign of fetal distress is the appearance of meconium (fetal bowel movement) in the amniotic fluid. Often it is meaningless, and in breech presentation, where the fetus's behind is squeezed, it can almost be expected that a bowel movement would occur. But in about 20 percent of cases, meconium denotes fetal distress, and the fetal monitor can provide a more detailed picture of what is going on.

Fetal monitors have gotten an undeserved reputation as the cause of unnecessary cesarean sections. There is definitely a limit at present to the technology; after all, the practitioner is attempting to define the status of the hidden patient (the fetus) by looking at one parameter—a pulse rate, and the effect of the contractions upon it. That is why pH studies can be so valuable to corroborate the information, as well as the clinical signs and the practitioner's good judgment.

Virtually all technology has the potential to be beneficial if used properly, or harmful if misused. Pregnant women and their practitioners have a marvelous tool at their disposal and should not shun it. The point of labor is to get the child born safely; fetal monitors can contribute to its successful accomplishment.

Q. *What can be given to me to reduce the pain of childbirth?*
Throughout pregnancy, one piece of advice remains constant: Avoid drugs wherever possible to reduce risks to the fetus,

unless your practitioner prescribes drugs that are necessary to your and the fetus's well-being.

By preparing you for labor and delivery and instructing you in breathing and other coping techniques, childbirth classes help diminish your need for anesthesia. In fact, many women who have drug-free labor and delivery feel a sense of personal triumph in their ability to withstand labor's challenges.

But you do not have to be a hero. No less an earth mother figure than the dancer Isadora Duncan proclaimed in her autobiography, "It is simply absurd that with our modern science painless childbirth does not exist as a *matter of course.* . . . Don't let me hear of any Woman's Movement or Sufragette Movement until women have put an end to this, I believe, wholly useless agony."

Following are the types of anesthesia used during labor and childbirth. Inform your practitioner if you have ever had allergic reaction to "-caine" drugs such as novocaine, lidocaine, or pontocaine, or to any other anesthetics.

- *Epidural anesthesia,* the injection of an anesthetic in a space at the base of the spinal cord, is a popular choice for both vaginal and cesarean delivery, because it enables you to be awake and pain-free for your baby's birth (an awesome sight you do not want to miss!). Epidurals numb your body below the umbilicus. If properly administered, the epidural usually does not impede childbirth, or harm or cause respiratory depression in the baby.
- *General anesthesia,* once a matter of course for many hospital births in the United States, today is less used during vaginal childbirth. It is used, however, for many cesarean sections, especially emergency C-sections when there is not time to administer an epidural. The practitioner must be aware of the risk of respiratory depression in the newborn.
- *Spinal block*—injection of an anesthetic directly into the

spinal fluid—is less frequently used because of the severe headaches it causes. The maternal blood pressure may fall significantly, compromising the blood supply and therefore the fetus's oxygen supply.

- *Pudendal block* involves an anesthetic administered through the vagina that numbs pudendal nerves supplying the vulvar area. It can be used primarily for forceps delivery or episiotomy.

Q. *Why might I need a cesarean section?*
Indications for cesarean section include:

- *Previous cesarean section*—"Once a C-section, always a C-section," a motto once meticulously followed, is no longer necessarily so. If the reason for the previous cesarean is not present in this pregnancy, and if the scar in the uterus is horizontal and in the lower uterine segment (as opposed to a "classical" vertical incision), then you can often attempt vaginal birth after cesarean (VBAC, pronounced vee-back). Do not assume, however, if your cesarean scar is a low horizontal "bikini cut," that the *uterine* scar is also horizontal; your practitioner must confirm what type of uterine scar you have. The force of labor may cause a classical incision to rupture, hence the need for repeat cesarean sections. Vertical incisions for cesarean sections are used in various circumstances, such as when the baby is not presenting in the normal fashion, or when the placenta is low, blocking the usual route of incision.
- *Failure of descent*—if the fetus does not descend through the cervix and birth canal, perhaps because it is too large to fit, then it must be delivered by cesarean.
- *Fetal distress*—when fetal monitoring and pH studies indicate that the fetus is acidotic and that its heart is having inappropriate responses to uterine contractions, i.e., bradycardia, which means a slow heartbeat. These factors

reveal that the fetus may not be able to survive the stress of vaginal delivery intact and healthy. Therefore, cesarean section is the safest course.

- *Placenta previa*—when the placenta, located low in the uterus, blocks the cervix. Cesarean is the only way for the baby to get out.
- *Abruptio placenta*—when the placenta disengages from the uterine wall, causing bleeding. An emergency cesarean is often necessary for the safety of both woman and child.
- *Labor fails to progress*—when the cervix does not dilate in an appropriate amount of time, or if the baby cannot engage in the pelvis, or if the cervix is fully dilated but the baby's head does not adequately descend, or rotate or flex properly, then a cesarean is needed.
- *Breech presentation*—when the fetus, instead of presenting headfirst, is turned so its leg(s) and buttocks face the cervix. Certain breech babies can be delivered vaginally, but cesarean delivery is safest for many types of breech.
- *Other abnormal presentations and lies,* such as transverse lie, when the baby's shoulder or side is presenting to the cervix, require cesarean section.
- *Multiple pregnancy.* Vaginal delivery is possible when twins are vertex-vertex (both have heads down), but if one twin is breech, a cesarean is needed to deliver both. The same applies to triplets, though the likelihood of delivering them (or quadruplets, etc.) vaginally is much smaller, since at least one is likely to be in breech position.
- *Herpes*—when the woman has active herpes lesions that could infect the baby if it were born vaginally.
- *Prolapsed umbilical cord*—when the umbilical cord descends through the vagina.

In some instances, such as breech presentation or multiple fetuses, you may know in advance that you will need a cesarean; in others, the cesarean will be a last-minute decision. Either way, cesarean often has an emotional as well as a physical impact. If you were really counting on having a vaginal birth, news that you need a cesarean can be a real blow. Your vision of the birth must now be altered. But cesarean is not second best; it is the *best* option for you at this time, for *this* baby's needs.

Whether you have a baby by cesarean or, as some doctors put it, "from below," the most important thing is having the baby safely and holding your healthy newborn in your arms. You did not "fail" to have vaginal birth—you *succeeded* in giving your child the best start in life.

CHAPTER 14

After the Baby Is Born

Q. *Should I breast-feed?*

Life turns inside-out when a fetus becomes a baby. It was inside, in fluid, floating in the dark; now it is out in the light, breathing the open air, encircled by your arms. But one thing can stay the same: It can still receive its nourishment just from you. The hardworking placenta has retired, but your breasts can provide the human equivalent of manna.

In *Fanny*, an eighteenth-century-style novel, Erica Jong described a new mother's experience:

> I'll ne'er forget, if I live to be a Hundred, how your little Mouth latch'd on to my Nipple as if there were nothing upon this whole Earth but Mouth and Breast, and all the Dance of Life were simply the Motion of an Infant's Lips, sucking, sucking, sucking!

While breast milk is universally acknowledged as the best nourishment for infants, the pleasure and loving exchange of breast-feeding are equally important reasons to nurse. Perhaps as additional incentives to breast-feeding, nature built in two "perks" for the mother: Breast-feeding helps your uterus contract to its former size, so you get your figure back sooner. And it is a natural form of birth control, reducing (though not completely eliminating) your likelihood of conceiving.

The composition of breast milk is tailor-made for babies; despite improved baby formula, even the baby-formula companies acknowledge that their products cannot equal the real thing.

Yet for some women there are compelling reasons *not* to breast-feed. And some women prefer a combination plan: breast-feeding in the morning and evening, for example, and bottle-feeding (or, in the case of working mothers, having a baby-sitter give a bottle) during the day.

The following chart compares breast-feeding and bottle-feeding. Make the choices that are best for *you*; the happier and more content you are, the happier your baby will be, too—whether fed by bottle or breast.

Advantages of Breast-feeding

Convenience
Your milk is always available—anytime, anywhere. It is easy to acquire the knack of discreet nursing, so you can breast-feed in public places. Wear loose tops over pants or skirts. A casual reach inside your collar will unfasten the flap of your nursing bra. Your clothing serves as a ready-made tent under which your baby can nurse. For extra modesty, lightly drape a shawl or receiving blanket over your shoulder.

Breast-feeding means no bottles to buy or clean up (except "relief bottles" if used).

Advantages of Bottle-feeding

Convenience
Disposable bottle liners and bottles and ready-mix infant formulas have made bottle-feeding more convenient than ever. While some mothers still like to use glass bottles, they should be sterilized prior to each use. And older babies, who sometimes announce that they've had enough by hurling bottles across the room, can cause a bit more damage with heavy glass bottles.

If you mix breast-feeding and bottle-feeding, you can express milk (and even freeze extra supplies for a few days) and have a baby-sitter give your baby a bottle filled with your own milk.

Nutritional Value

Breast milk is truly one of nature's wonders. It is a great example of a supply-and-demand commodity: Your body supplies what the baby demands. (Provided, of course, that you are eating well and drinking enough fluids.) No infant formula can match the many components of breast milk— among which are antibodies the mother passes on to her baby. These lessen the likelihood that the infant will become sick in that crucial, vulnerable first part of life.

Breast milk is highly digestible, which means your baby will be far less likely to be constipated or have diarrhea or gas.

The Exercise of Sucking

Breast-feeding requires that the baby suck harder than it would need to with a bottle. But don't feel sorry for putting baby up to this task. The effort the baby expends is really fine exercise, and helps in the formation of its developing palate, jaw, and teeth. A "good sucking baby," to use one nurse's favorite compliment, will benefit from its daily workouts.

Nutritional Value

No one pretends that infant formula is breast milk's nutritional equal. Nor, however, is it analogous to a poor relation. Millions of babies raised on infant formula have thrived beautifully. In fact, when breast-feeding fell out of fashion in the 1950s and 1960s, nearly all babies were bottle-fed and did fine. You have more choices of infant formula today, including soy-based formulas for infants who are allergic to cow's milk. If you choose to bottle-feed your baby, chances are that it will grow up just as healthy as a breast-fed child.

The Exercise of Sucking

Seek out nipples (and, if you use them, pacifiers) that are shaped to exercise your baby's mouth and jaw. Look for labels that describe the product as being similar to the breast-feeding experience.

Getting Your Figure Back
Nursing your baby means
expending hundreds of calories
that *you* don't need on your own
body! Some of your baby's
nutrients will come from the
food you eat and milk and other
fluids you drink. But others will
be drawn from fat stored by your
body during pregnancy. If you
eat a well-balanced diet, and
avoid excess fats, sweets, and
"empty" calories, nursing your
baby will help you lose
pregnancy weight faster.

Getting Dad Involved
Breast-feeding creates priceless
moments for mother and baby—
intimate hours lying side by side
or musing in a rocking chair.
But what about Dad? There are
several ways to make sure he
does not feel left out.
Occasionally, express milk and
let him give it to the baby in a
bottle (perhaps while you take a
break and go out to a movie
with a friend). If you choose not
to use any bottles, he can still
bathe the baby, walk and rock
it, and feed it once it begins to
take solids.

Sensual Considerations
Many women consider breast-
feeding one of the greatest

Getting Your Figure Back
Bottle-feeding mothers do not
have to keep up their pregnancy
diet and can eat less than breast-
feeding mothers. So if you are
determined to lose pregnancy
weight fast, you can choose a
well-balanced diet without
having to think about whether it
contains enough nutrients for
both you and your baby.

Getting Dad Involved
Bottle-feeding means that both
mother and father can equally
nourish the baby, holding the
baby close during feedings; it is
so satisfying to see the baby
being satisfied.

Many men appreciate feeling
self-sufficient with the baby; it is
not only the mother who can
meet the baby's needs, but Dad,
too. This also gives the mother
much more freedom.

Sensual Considerations
As satisfying as breast-feeding
can be for many women, that's

sensual pleasures of their lives. They feel proud that they can nourish the baby as well after birth as they did during pregnancy. But it is not only an altruistic activity. Nothing can compare with stretching out on a bed, your baby lying beside you nursing, then falling asleep together. The nipple stimulation of breast-feeding feels wonderful and promotes a womanly feeling of peace and contentment that many women treasure with all their hearts.

how much of a turnoff it can be for others. Not every woman is comfortable with handling or exposing her breasts, and some women find even "discreet" nursing in public never discreet enough. And not every woman wants to have that particular physical connection with her baby. One woman said, "I spent nine months pregnant. Now I want my body back." Sometimes a woman *wants* to nurse but simply cannot feel relaxed doing it. If she is tense, her milk often will not flow well, which makes the baby tense, too. So what is the point of continuing to breast-feed? If you are a happier person when you are bottle-feeding, then your baby will be, too.

Q.   *If I breast-feed, how do I care for my breasts?*

- *Wear a nursing bra that gives good support.* Your breasts are larger and heavier now. A good bra prevents your breasts from drooping and reduces the likelihood of lasting stretch marks. Check out different styles of nursing bras to see which will be most convenient for you. Some clasps can be unfastened with one hand, a real advantage if you are holding a crying baby in the other.

    If milk leaks from your breasts, buy nursing pads to tuck inside your bra to catch the leaks.
- *Keep nipples supple by avoiding soaps and petroleum jelly.*

Nipples are kept moist by their own natural oils and perspiration. Wash them with water only. If your nipples are very dry or cracked, a simple lanolin cream can help. So will exposing nipples to the air frequently.

- *Nursing regularly keeps milk flowing and your breasts comfortable.* One evening you decide to go out for dinner with a friend, which means you will skip breast-feeding the baby. You leave a bottle with your husband or baby-sitter and take off for a much-needed break. But your breasts have their own "built-in clock." Around the time you would normally breast-feed, you will feel the "letdown reflex," a tingly, heavy sensation that announces that milk has accumulated in your breasts, ready for the baby to suck. You can't really just ignore it, because in just a few hours your breasts will become hard and engorged. You have several solutions:

1. Express milk before you go out for the evening. Use a manual or electric breast pump, or develop the knack of expressing milk without a pump. (Stroke your breasts a few times toward the nipple to stimulate milk flow. Hold your right nipple between the thumb and forefinger of your right hand. Press your fingers in so you can feel the ribs behind your breasts, and squeeze your nipple rhythmically, expressing milk into a clean bottle or cup. Repeat with the left breast and hand.) If you have not expressed enough milk, or are out later than you expected and your breasts become engorged, you can always excuse yourself to go to the rest room and express a bit of milk to give yourself some relief.

2. Tolerate the fullness in your breasts and nurse the baby as soon as you get home. Make sure you let your husband or baby-sitter know of your plan, so they will not feed your baby just before you get there! You want

the baby to be hungry for your milk. Don't worry if
the baby is asleep. Many a woman, eager for breast
relief, has rushed into her home, not even bothering
to take off her coat, and scooped up her sleepy baby
from the crib, plopped into a rocking chair, and awak-
ened the baby just enough to nurse. Babies are usually
very cooperative—and mothers are very grateful. It
is a perfect illustration of the symbiosis of nursing.

3. If you plan to go out often, or if you just want to build
in an hour or so for yourself every evening, you may
have your partner give the baby a bottle every evening
(reserving the late-night feeding for yourself). For
many fathers, regular responsibility for one feeding
promotes bonding with the infant and gives them an
opportunity to help you. Your breasts will adjust to
the new schedule (and adjust that amazing built-in
clock) so you will not become engorged.

*Vary your breast-feeding position so that your nipples are not
always pressed in the same place.* Experiment with different nursing
positions both sitting up and lying down.

*Consult your practitioner if one or both breasts becomes red, hot,
and tender, and if you have a fever.* These are symptoms of breast
infection. Warm soaks and an antibiotic usually take care of the
problem quickly. When infections are severe and persistent, you
may need to stop breast-feeding. But most women are able to
continue nursing even through the infection, especially if they
only have the infection in one breast, and certainly afterward.

Q. *What should I expect while recuperating?*
You may feel so elated by your baby's birth that you could
leap among the clouds. But your body is by no means ready for
such exertion! Labor is very hard work, and you need to allow
yourself time to rest afterward. And you need to adjust to a
number of changes:

Hormonal changes affecting body and emotions begin virtually the moment the baby is born. Hormones that supported the pregnancy are no longer needed, while those that support breast-feeding come into play. This hormonal rearranging helps your uterus begin the process of returning to normal and prepares your breasts to produce colostrum (the clear liquid breasts produce for the three days or so before the milk "comes in").

This time of transition between pregnancy and "back to normal" can wreak havoc with your emotions. "Postpartum depression" is a mix of crying jags and mood swings that some women experience for ten days or more after giving birth. While hormonal changes certainly carry some of the blame for this upset, it is also due in part to the fact that having a baby represents a major life upheaval. As much as you want this baby, you are also thrust into a new and highly responsible role, a new sleep pattern (if you are lucky enough to get any!), and a revised relationship with your partner (and any older children you may have). Add the tensions of family squabbles over what to name the baby, calls from your office inquiring when you'll be back, having to plan for the baby's homecoming, the prospect of writing fifty thank-you notes for baby gifts, and the messiness of closets you never had a chance to clean while you were pregnant (and certainly won't get to now), and you have the makings of a postpartum cocktail—similar to Molotov, but longer-lasting.

But many women never experience postpartum depression. If you are among those who do, it will most likely subside after ten days to two weeks. To help get you through it, you might find it helpful to imagine that you have a Good-Witch-Glinda bubble around you that gently but firmly repels any tensions. Within the bubble, hold and feed your baby, embrace your partner, cuddle and read to your older children, chat on the phone only with people who make you feel good, eat delicious healthy foods, and drink fresh juices. Set this time apart from all else, to ease out of pregnancy and into motherhood.

If depression is severe, you may need psychiatric help. If

depression is mild but lingers beyond a couple of weeks, you might benefit from the support of a new mothers' group (ask your pediatrician to recommend one).

Breast-feeding is an instinctual skill for baby, a learned one for you. Maternity nurses are accustomed to the sight of a husband reading aloud from a breast-feeding manual while his wife follows directions about how to shift the baby into different breast-feeding positions. Transforming you and your baby into a happy nursing couple is an absorbing project that will occupy you for several days after delivery—but once you get the hang of it, nursing will feel natural and easy.

If you choose not to nurse, your practitioner might prescribe hormonal supplements to suppress milk. But this is not usually necessary, since breasts will engorge, then naturally go back to their nonnursing state.

Episiotomy, while technically a minor surgery, can present major feelings of discomfort. Ice packs on your perineum for the first twenty-four hours after delivery help keep swelling down. After that, you can obtain some relief from warm sitz baths or compresses. Keep the perineum clean by squirting it with warm water from a squeeze bottle after urinating or bowel movements. Change sanitary pads every few hours.

Sometimes women fear that the stitches will rip out when they have a bowel movement—so they postpone defecating and become constipated. Not to worry—the stitches will hold fast. An enema is not usually necessary to get your bowels moving again.

Sitting will be uncomfortable until stitches heal (in a week or two). So recline on your side, or sit on an inflatable "doughnut," available at medical-supply stores. The doughnut suspends your perineum slightly over the chair or bed, so there is no pressure on the stitches.

* * *

Cesarean-section Delivery. Recuperation occurs in several stages. For the first few days after the cesarean, you will need pain medication. Your practitioner can prescribe pain medication that will not interfere with breast-feeding. Applying supportive pressure to your abdomen when you sneeze or cough also aids recovery.

Many women's complaints of intense pain can be attributed to "gas." The "gas" pain comes from the fact that the abdominal cavity is entered and the bowel becomes paralyzed for a time; once peristalsis resumes, the gas is passed.

Protect the abdomen from strain by holding a pillow to your abdomen when you cough, laugh, sneeze, have a bowel movement, or in any way change position. Doing a breathing exercise with the pillow speeds return of good muscle tone: While hugging the pillow, slowly inhale through your nose, then press the pillow gently against you while you exhale through your mouth.

Pillows also come in handy when breast-feeding. When holding the baby, rest your arms on a pillow for support. And use another pillow as a "shield" on your incision. Newborn babies look fragile, but they kick with karate power. After you receive a kick to the abdomen, you will have a great deal of respect for your infant's strength—and a strong motivation to remember the pillow!

The day after your operation, it is time for your first walk, though it is the last thing you feel like doing. But with support from your partner or nurse, meet the challenge. Sitting up, dangling legs at the side of the bed, and then getting up for a brief stroll will aid circulation and healing. With each walk, tortoise-slow as it may be, you will feel your strength increase. You will probably feel tempted to hunch over to protect your incision, but trying to stay as regally straight as possible is actually much better—not only for your blood circulation and healing, but also for your state of mind.

A few days after your cesarean, you can probably take a shower (not a bath). Because you may feel dizzy occasionally while standing, have your partner or a nurse stand by while you are in the shower and help you back to bed afterward.

Your doctor will probably remove stitches or staples just before you check out. Once home, get plenty of rest, move about slowly, do breathing exercises, and concentrate on enjoying your baby and on getting your strength back.

Q.   *Should I request rooming-in?*

Rooming-in—having your baby with you instead of in the nursery—gives you more time together, lets you nurse on demand, and enables the baby to have plenty of skin-to-skin contact with Mom instead of being alone in a nursery crib. Yet rooming-in does have some drawbacks. You may feel exhausted and unable to care for your baby full time right away. You may simply need some time for yourself—not only to sleep, but to spend time with your partner, with older children, with close family and friends, or simply alone. In the nursery, a baby can be well cared for and can sleep perfectly comfortably—so you can sleep deeply, unworried about having to listen for the baby's stirrings.

Rooming-in does not have to be an all-or-nothing choice. Many hospitals permit flexible rooming-in, so you can have the baby with you all day but in the nursery at night. Or you can have the option to decide at any time during the day or night whether to have your baby with you. When you go home, you will probably not have the luxury of being able to claim time alone when you want it. So flexible rooming-in may be just the right choice for you.

Whatever you decide, make sure you base your choice on what is right for you—not on what you feel you "should" do.

Q.   *Is it okay for visitors to hold or get close to the baby?*

Hospitals differ in their policies. Some require that all babies, even those who are rooming in, stay in the nursery during visiting hours, while others permit guests to don sterile gowns and hold the new infant. Naturally, you would not want anyone who is ill to hold the baby or visit you.

Q. My religion does not require circumcision of male infants. Should I have my baby boy circumcised anyway?

Circumcision is an optional surgical procedure, with pros and cons. Among circumcision's benefits:

- Circumcision protects against phimosis, a painful (though uncommon) condition involving the foreskin.
- If a child's father, brothers, and other family members and friends are circumcised, he will not want to look different.

Among its drawbacks:

- Circumcision, like any operative procedure, however minor, can have complications (such as infection or urethral injury).
- Some people believe that the procedure causes psychological trauma (though proponents of circumcision believe the infant actually feels little pain).

Q. How long must we stay in the hospital?

The usual stay for a vaginal birth is decreasing rapidly. Presently it may be two or three days or even less; for a cesarean, a maximum of four or five days, barring complications. The hospital stay enables you to rest and recuperate and gives the pediatric staff an opportunity to observe the baby. In particular, they look for signs of jaundice, a fairly common condition in which the baby's skin acquires a yellowish hue. Jaundice is caused by excess amounts of bilirubin, a breakdown product of red blood cells. Usually, the jaundice will go away by itself. Many babies with mild cases are exposed to ultraviolet light (with their eyes protected), and the condition disappears within a day or two. If jaundice peaks at very high levels, the baby may need an exchange transfusion of blood in order to lower the level of bilirubin and protect the baby's brain from damage.

CHAPTER 15

At Home Again

Q. How can I help siblings adjust to the new baby?

Try to include children in preparing for the baby and in caring for it afterward. Take them on shopping trips and let them select the baby's new undershirts—and a stuffed toy that will be their personal gift to the new baby. Many hospitals permit siblings to visit their mother and the new baby. It may be wise to have the baby in the nursery when siblings visit, so they can first reunite with you and have all your attention to themselves. Then you can go to the nursery together to see the baby. In subsequent visits, let them hold the baby (with your support).

At home, even the youngest siblings can be helpful. They can gently stroke the baby when it is crying or sing a lullaby, hold a bottle, or lightly tap the baby's back to help it burp. They feel important when asked to fetch a diaper or a blanket—but remember that many young children are attached to their baby blankets, even those that are not the "special one." If possible, buy the baby its own blankets.

Whether you breast-feed or bottle-feed, the baby's mealtime is a great opportunity to cuddle with an older child and read a story or look at drawings. When the baby naps, you should nap, too—and perhaps your older child can lie down with you. As busy as you will be with the new baby, apply your ingenuity to finding time to spend with your older children individually and together. Even five minutes of your undivided attention can mean the world to a little child.

Help older children bond with the new baby by interpreting the baby's actions in a positive way: "Look, the baby is watching you. She admires how her big brother can jump." Or, "See how the baby holds your finger so tight? He loves you."

When siblings express dislike of the baby, it is usually a signal that they need hugs and reassurances of your love: "I know the baby cries a lot. When it is big like you, it will know how to ask for things by talking. I am so proud of how big you are, but you are still my baby, too, you know." Show siblings photos of their own babyhood, pointing out how you also fed and diapered them.

Q. *How soon can I have sex after having the baby?*

Sex should be avoided until your reproductive tract's natural barriers to infection are restored. That is, when the cervix is fully closed, the uterus involuted, the episiotomy scar healed. After examining you, your practitioner can tell you when you can resume sexual relations.

Breast-feeding women often find sex uncomfortable at first because of vaginal dryness. Try using a lubricant such as K-Y Jelly.

Q. *What contraception should I use when we resume sexual relations? Do I need to use contraception if I am breast-feeding?*

Breast-feeding does suppress ovulation and menstruation, but it cannot be relied upon as a foolproof method of birth control. So when you resume sexual relations, use barrier methods—a diaphragm, or a condom, which is especially effective when used in conjunction with contraceptive foam. Avoid birth-control pills, however, since the hormones they contain may be passed to your baby through breast milk. If you are bottle-feeding, birth-control pills should not pose a problem if your practitioner believes that you are a good candidate for their use. If you smoke, you should try to stop if you plan to use birth control pills because of the somewhat increased risk of stroke.

Q. What postpartum medical care do I need?

Most practitioners advise you to have a checkup six weeks after delivery. By that time, your uterus has shrunk down to its normal size, a process called *involution*, and your weight loss will likely be under way.

There is a lot to talk about at the six-week checkup:

Diet. If you are breast-feeding, continue the pregnancy diet, making sure you drink enough milk and water. Through the six weeks after delivery, continue taking prenatal vitamin supplements; at the checkup, ask whether to continue. Usually, vitamin and iron supplements are recommended for nursing mothers.

If you are bottle-feeding, you may want to request a balanced weight-loss plan. Do not try to rush weight loss—you need your energy to continue recuperation and to take care of your baby. But by eating high-quality foods, cutting back on fat and sugar, and getting enough exercise (including taking the baby out for a daily stroll), you should be able to shed pregnancy pounds easily.

Exercise. Ask your practitioner about recommended exercises; if you have had a cesarean, make sure you do not put stress on the abdominal incision.

The exercises described in this book for pregnancy are also effective for postpartum toning. Now that you can do exercises on your back, you can add the "bicycle" (pedaling in the air while in a shoulder stand) and straight leg raises (lying on your back and raising and lowering each leg in turn, and then both together).

This is also a good time to begin doing Kegel exercises to tone vaginal, vulvar, and urethral muscles; a companion exercise, the "buttock press," helps tone sphincter muscles. After childbirth, the elasticity of the "between the legs" muscles can diminish, with disconcerting results. You might become slightly incontinent, unable to keep urine from dribbling out on your way to the bathroom.

Kegel exercises are effective and easy, even pleasurable to do—and they are invisible. You can stand at a bus stop tightening vaginal or anal muscles, and no one will know but you. Improved vaginal tone can also improve sex: Your ability to rhythmically massage your partner's penis with your internal muscles heightens sexual pleasure for both of you.

How to Do Kegel Exercises

When you urinate, try to stop the flow of the urine. You will feel your muscles tighten. Then let the flow resume, and stop it again. Do this every time you urinate. At first you may not be able to stop the flow, then you may feel the flow diminish somewhat, and eventually you will be able to "turn it on and off" with your new muscle power. To do the buttock press, simply tighten buttock muscles so they feel hard and clenched, then relax. You will notice the sphincter muscles closing tighter. When you are more accustomed to locating the sphincter muscles, you can do the exercise more subtly, without tightening the entire buttock area.

Now that you are in touch with those muscles, find other opportunities to tighten, then relax them: While you are doing dishes, sorting the mail, waiting in line at the bank, and during your regular exercise routine.

Adjustment to Motherhood. Many women use the six-week checkup as a time to confide the pleasures and problems of adjusting to their new role. It is often reassuring to know that it is quite common to feel exhausted, frustrated, and overwhelmed— in addition to proud, happy, and increasingly competent. You may want to ask your practitioner (or your childbirth-class

teacher) about a playgroup you might join or organize. It may
sound odd—a playgroup for babies who do not yet really play.
But such groups are for the mothers' benefit as much as the
babies', and as the children grow, they have a ready-made group
of playmates.

CHAPTER 16

The Conclusion:
A Beginning

The best piece of advice anyone can give a new mother is: Enjoy your baby. Even on frustrating days, or during endless nights of crying and rocking, remember that childhood is, on balance, a fleeting moment. Treasure it. Grab opportunities here and there to keep a journal of your child's accomplishments. Take lots of pictures. Go out for daily walks; hold your baby in your lap on a park bench and listen to birds sing and watch older children play. Before too long, that will be your baby grown up enough to sit on the swing, climb the jungle gym . . . walk on the balance beam, *stand* on the swing . . . baby-sit for small babies . . . become a parent. Pregnancy was a nine-month rainbow, and these are the golden moments that awaited you at its end.

Enjoy them.

Index

About the Authors

Ronald M. Caplan, M.D., C.M., is Clinical Associate Professor, Obstetrics and Gynecology, Cornell University Medical College, and Attending Obstetrician/Gynecologist at the New York Hospital. He is a Fellow of the American College of Obstetricians and Gynecologists, the American College of Surgeons, and the Royal College of Surgeons of Canada, and is a member of the Society of Reproductive Surgeons, the American Fertility Society, and other medical organizations. He is the editor of *Advances in Obstetrics and Gynecology* (Williams and Wilkins, 1978), *Principles of Obstetrics* (Williams and Wilkins, 1982), *Pregnant Is Beautiful* (Pocket Books/Simon & Schuster, 1981), and *The Doctor's Guide to Pregnancy Over Thirty* (Ballantine Books, 1986), and has contributed to various other books and articles in the field. He has appeared on *The Today Show* and other television programs, and has been quoted in many periodicals as an expert on reproductive health. He is in private practice in Manhattan.

Betty Rothbart, M.S.W., is a health/science writer and educator in New York. She received a B.A. degree in English Education and Theatre Arts, and a Master of Social Work degree from the University of Pittsburgh. She is the author of *Frontiers in Fertility* (Planned Parenthood Federation of America) and co-author of *Hemorrhoids* (Consumer Reports Books), *Hernias* (Consumer Reports Books), and other health books and articles. She is the major writer of HIV/AIDS curriculum for the New York City schools, and is currently writing a book about parenting twins, to be published by William Morrow. She has taught writing at Hunter College's School of Health Sciences and has lectured about HIV/AIDS education at the Bank Street College of Education. She is a member of the American Society of Journalists and Authors, the Author's Guild, and the Society of Children's Book Writers.